Physical Principles and Clinical Applications of Nuclear Magnetic Resonance

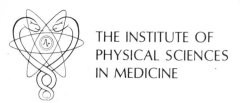

THE INSTITUTE OF
PHYSICAL SCIENCES
IN MEDICINE

Physical Principles and Clinical Applications of Nuclear Magnetic Resonance

Edited by R A Lerski

IPSM 2

© The Hospital Physicists' Association 1985
47 Belgrave Square
London SW1X 8QX

ISBN 0 904181 38 3

HᵥH 7716 /25 20 1·92

Manufactured in Great Britain by
Paradigm Print, Gateshead

Contents

Introduction

In the space of less than three years the applications of Nuclear Magnetic Resonance (NMR) in medicine have blossomed from laboratory curiosity to the source of intense commercial activity and remarkable clinical results. Installations of imaging equipment proceed at breakneck pace with image quality rivalling the best of x-ray computerized tomography. In parallel, the new field of Topical Magnetic Resonance (TMR) promises the disclosure of a whole host of biochemical information *in vivo*.

This speed of development and the fact that much of the best results have been achieved under the cloak of commercial secrecy have made it difficult for those interested in the field to become acquainted with its intricacies. The present text represents an attempt to ease this problem and has grown out of papers presented at a joint Hospital Physicists' Association and Institution of Electrical Engineers meeting held in London on 5 May 1983.

Invited papers by leading UK experts in NMR are intended to cover NMR imaging from basic principles, through magnet design, electronics systems and reconstruction methods to clinical results, and TMR in both technical and clinical aspects.

Many basic questions remain to be answered in NMR with regard to the equipment parameters for the optimal clinical results. Perhaps the most critical of these, certainly in terms of capital cost, is the best static field for an imaging system. While the basic signal to noise in NMR increases at least linearly with static field many other factors influence the final image signal-to-noise and at the time of writing it is not at all established that imaging at fields around 1 tesla is likely to be best. T_1 contrast is not constant with magnetic field and there is some evidence that lower fields (~ 0.1 T) may provide the optimal discrimination between tissue types. The absolute value of T_1 tends to increase with field so that although theoretically an improved signal-to-noise should allow a reduced scanning time for fixed resolution, in practice this will not be the case.

Receiver coil design and interference screening in imaging systems are probably not optimal and substantial gains may be possible in these areas. A wealth of clever techniques developed in experimental pulse NMR have not yet been applied to either imaging or TMR.

Finally, what distinguishes NMR from x-ray computerized tomography or ultrasound and may in the end be its greatest strength is the potential to make quantitative measurement of either tissue water behaviour or phosphorus metabolism.

The next three years promise further exciting advances and progress in the following years can only be guessed at.

R A Lerski
London, 1984

CHAPTER 1 **Principles of nuclear magnetic resonance**

W Vennart

Department of Physics, University of Exeter,
Exeter, England

1.1. Introduction

1.1.1. Basic physics

The hydrogen atom is present extensively in the human body, in water, and in biological molecules such as proteins. This introductory chapter on nuclear magnetic resonance (NMR) will be confined to the NMR properties of the nucleus of the hydrogen atom—the proton.

The proton can be considered essentially as a sphere of positive charge which spins on its axis. This circulating charge gives rise to a current loop that endows the proton with a magnetic moment and it behaves, therefore, like a tiny bar magnet. When a system of protons (a human subject, for example) is immersed in a large static magnetic field (approximately 1 tesla, 1 T), the magnetic moments of the protons interact with the field and precess around it. Some of the protons precess with their axes pointing in the same direction as the field and some against it. This precession is analogous to the way in which a gyroscope precesses in the Earth's gravitational field; it too can align itself with its axis pointing either vertically up or down.

If radiofrequency radiation (the frequency of which is determined by the magnitude of the static magnetic field) is incident upon the protons then it can induce them to change from precessing with the magnetic field to against it, or vice versa. In equilibrium in the static magnetic field (no radiofrequency radiation present) the number of protons precessing in the same direction as the field is slightly more than those oppositely directed, because the former is the lower energy state. There is thus a small net magnetization pointing in the direction of the static magnetic field. When radiofrequency radiation is applied to the sample, more protons, therefore, are elevated to the higher energy state (precessing against the field) by absorption of energy, than give up energy by being stimulated to transfer into the lower energy state (precessing with the field). The proton system thus absorbs radiofrequency radiation and this can be detected by standard techniques. The intensity of the signal detected depends on the number of protons present and its character depends on their chemical environment.

After the radiofrequency radiation has been switched off, the system of protons reverts back to its equilibrium configuration by various relaxation mechanisms whose time constants (which are typically of the order of tens of milliseconds) can be measured. These time constants are governed by the physical and chemical environment of the protons and can give information about the dynamics and structure of the molecules in which the protons are embedded.

This then is the basis of the NMR experiment. The following sections are intended to supplement the simple picture outlined above.

1.1.2. Current techniques

In their early work Bloch *et al.*[1, 2] demonstrated that the NMR signals from materials could be obtained in several ways, in particular by continuous wave and pulse techniques. First employed were continuous wave methods in which the sample under investigation is immersed in a high magnetic field that can be swept about a central value while the sample is irradiated with radio-frequency radiation—the NMR spectrum is then obtained continuously. With the advent of new technologies, pulse techniques (in which the transient behaviour of the nuclei in a sample immersed in a high magnetic field is measured after they have been disturbed by a short burst of radiofrequency radiation) became more widely used. This latter technique obtains the NMR spectrum more quickly and is more versatile; consequently NMR imaging machines and nearly all modern NMR research equipment employ pulsed NMR systems. The basic ideas behind pulsed NMR techniques will be discussed in this chapter, with some reference to continuous wave methods to illustrate fundamental concepts.

1.2. Nuclear magnetism

1.2.1. Classical model

The proton possesses a positive charge and intrinsic spin angular momentum which combine to give it a magnetic dipole moment. From this classical mechanics viewpoint a proton with magnetic moment μ will experience a torque when immersed in a magnetic field B_0 inclined at angle θ, figure 1(a). The rate of change of the angular momentum J is given by

$$\mu \wedge B_0 = \frac{dJ}{dt} \tag{1}$$

where $\wedge$ indicates the vector cross product.

It can be seen from this equation that the proton will precess about the applied field in a direction perpendicular to the plane μ and B_0 (in the case of figure 1(a) out of the plane of the diagram). The rotational frequency (ω_0) of this precession can be derived by considering the small changes of the

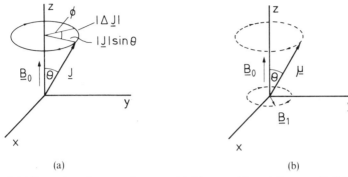

(a)   (b)

Figure 1. (a) Precession of a magnetic moment (μ) immersed in a static magnetic field B_0 and (b) with an additional rotating magnetic field (B_1) applied.

angular momentum $|\Delta J|$ as the proton rotates about B_0 (figure 1(a)). In a time Δt, J will precess through an angle ϕ given by

$$\phi = |\omega_0|\Delta t$$

and will change by an amount $|\Delta J|$ given by

$$|\Delta J| = |J|\sin\theta . \phi$$

Substituting for ϕ from above we get

$$|\Delta J| = |J|\sin\theta |\omega_0|\Delta t$$

In the limit of small $|\Delta J|$ and Δt this equation can be written in the differential form

$$\frac{d|J|}{dt} = |J|\sin\theta|\omega_0| \tag{2}$$

Substituting for $d|J|/dt$ from equation (1) we have

$$\mu \wedge B_0 = |J|\sin\theta|\omega_0|$$

By expanding the cross product we get

$$|\mu||B_0|\sin\theta = |J|\sin\theta|\omega_0|$$

and hence

$$|\omega_0| = \frac{|\mu||B_0|}{|J|}$$

or

$$|\omega_0| = \gamma|B_0| \tag{3}$$

where γ = gyromagnetic ratio = $\dfrac{\text{magnetic moment}}{\text{angular momentum}}$.

1.2.2. Quantum mechanical model

From the theory of quantum mechanics it is found that a proton with spin I and magnetic moment μ immersed in a magnetic field B_0 can only assume certain discrete orientations within that field (figure 2). The length of the nuclear angular momentum vector is $[I(I+1)]^{1/2}\hbar$, however the only measurable components of this vector are given by $m_I\hbar$ where m_I, the magnetic quantum number, can take any of $(2I+1)$ values $m_I = I,(I-1)\ldots-(I-1)$, $-I$. Thus for the proton with $I = 1/2$ there will be just two orientations that

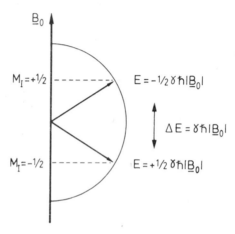

Figure 2. Orientation of a spin 1/2 nucleus, in this case a proton, in a magnetic field B_0 along the z-direction. The spacing of the two energy levels is indicated on the diagram.

it can assume in a magnetic field B_0 (figure 2) and two measurable values of I and hence μ_I. It should be noted that usually only derived or measured values of the projection of μ are quoted as the magnetic moment since this is the only value of interest experimentally. For the proton, therefore, in a magnetic field B_0 there will be two energy levels (corresponding to the two orientations it can assume with respect to the field), i.e., one with its spin directed parallel to the field (low energy state) and the other with its spin oppositely directed (high energy state); see figure 2. The energy of these two states is given by

$$E = -\mu.B = -\gamma\hbar m_I |B_0|$$

where in this case, for protons, $m_I = \pm 1/2$.

At room temperature there is a slightly greater probability of finding a proton in the lower energy state rather than in the higher state (as will be shown later). Transitions between the two states can take place if the quantum mechanical selection rule that m_I changes by ± 1 is obeyed. Thus the change in energy of the proton in going from one state to the other is $\Delta E = \gamma\hbar|B_0|$;

in other words, for a proton to be excited from the lower energy state (spinning with the field) to the upper state (spinning against the field) requires an exact quantum of energy to be absorbed, given by

$$\hbar|\omega_0| = \gamma\hbar|\boldsymbol{B}_0|$$
$$|\omega_0| = \gamma|\boldsymbol{B}_0| \tag{4}$$

It should be noted that equations (3) and (4) are identical; the former was derived from classical mechanics and the latter from quantum mechanics. The main difference between the two approaches is that the angular momentum classically ($\boldsymbol{J}$) becomes quantized in the quantum mechanical formulation in units of $I\hbar$. From quantum mechanics it is found that electromagnetic radiation with its magnetic vector circularly polarized in the plane perpendicular to the static magnetic field ($\boldsymbol{B}_0$) is required to induce transitions between the two levels. For the classical case it is clear (figure 1(b)) that just such a condition must be met if a magnetic dipole is to change its orientation (θ) with respect to $\boldsymbol{B}_0$. This condition is achieved when a magnetic field, $\boldsymbol{B}_1$ (associated with the incident electromagnetic radiation) rotates at the resonant frequency (ω_0) about $\boldsymbol{B}_0$. Only then will the dipole experience a synchronized couple $\boldsymbol{\mu} \wedge \boldsymbol{B}_1$ tending to increase θ.

If $\boldsymbol{B}_1$ rotates at a different frequency then it will only produce small perturbations to the motion of the magnetic dipole. There is, therefore, good agreement between classical and quantum mechanical results (this is further elaborated in references 3 and 4) and this enables one to view many of the NMR phenomena from a "classical" viewpoint, and consequently to obtain a clear physical picture of NMR experiments.

1.3. Experimental considerations

It can be seen from equations (3) and (4) that the resonant frequency of the radiofrequency radiation, necessary to produce transitions between the two proton energy levels, changes with applied magnetic field $\boldsymbol{B}_0$. For protons in a magnetic field of 1 T the resonant frequency is 42.6 MHz (phosphorus-31 in a field would have a resonant frequency of 17.2 MHz). NMR experiments are usually carried out using static magnetic fields of the order of 1 T because these fields are fairly easy to achieve experimentally and, as will be seen later, the signal-to-noise ratio improves with increasing field.

If a system of protons, such as a sample of water, is immersed in a magnetic field and it is assumed that there is only weak coupling between the individual protons, then they will distribute themselves between the two energy levels described previously. The relative populations of the two levels will be given by the Boltzmann Distribution:

$$\frac{n\uparrow}{n\downarrow} = \exp\frac{\Delta E}{kT_\mathrm{S}} \tag{5}$$

where $n\uparrow$ = number of protons oriented parallel to $\boldsymbol{B}_0$, i.e., $m_I = +1/2$ state,
$\quad n\downarrow$ = number of protons oriented antiparallel to $\boldsymbol{B}_0$, i.e., $m_I = -1/2$ state,
$\quad k$ = Boltzmann constant
$\quad T_S$ = absolute temperature of the spin system—this will equal the lattice temperature T_L when the sample is in equilibrium,
$\quad \Delta E$ = energy splitting between the two levels, i.e., $\gamma\hbar|\boldsymbol{B}_0|$.

(Note that to describe relaxation processes it is usual to assign a spin temperature T_S to the proton spin system and a lattice temperature T_L to the system in which the spins are embedded; in the example above the lattice is the bulk water. In equilibrium the temperatures of the lattice and spin systems are equal.)

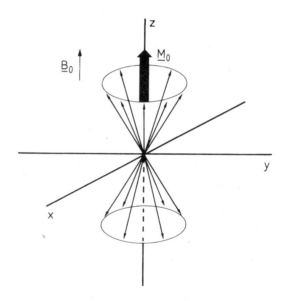

Figure 3. Precession of an assembly of protons in a magnetic field $\boldsymbol{B}_0$ giving rise to a net magnetization $\boldsymbol{M}_0$ in the z-direction.

At room temperature in a magnetic field of 1 T $n\uparrow/n\downarrow \sim 1 + 4 \times 10^{-6}$ for protons; thus there is a small net magnetization, $\boldsymbol{M}_0$, in the direction of the static magnetic field $\boldsymbol{B}_0$. It is this magnetization, which is the difference between the magnetic moments aligned with the field and those against it (figure 3), that is detected in NMR experiments. It is usual to consider $\boldsymbol{M}_0$ rotating at the Larmor frequency, ω_0, when one envisages the NMR experiment. From equation (5) it can be seen that as $\boldsymbol{B}_0$ increases $\boldsymbol{M}_0$ increases and thus the signal-to-noise ratio will increase.

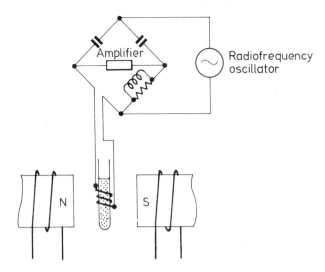

Figure 4. Schematic diagram of a system for obtaining a continuous wave NMR spectrum.

In the simple case of a continuous wave experiment, schematically represented in figure 4, the sample is immersed in a static magnetic field, B_0, and then irradiated with radiofrequency radiation (frequency ω_0) perpendicular to B_0 through a solenoid wound around the sample. The field B_0 is then slowly swept from $|B_0| - |\Delta B_0|$ to $|B_0| + |\Delta B_0|$, i.e., from below to above the resonant condition $|\omega_0| = \gamma |B_0|$. At resonance the sample will absorb radiation, which will cause an imbalance in the bridge circuit.

An absorption of radiation will take place because at resonance protons will be stimulated either to emit energy by making transitions from $m_I = -1/2$ to $m_I = +1/2$, or to absorb energy by the transition $m_I = +1/2$ to $m_I = -1/2$. These two transition rates are equal, but since there is an excess of protons in the lower energy state (equation (5)) there will be a net absorption of energy. Typically, a Lorentzian shaped absorption curve is obtained from a sample of water (figure 5(a)). It has finite width due to several parameters. One factor leading to this broadening is that the static magnetic field will not be uniform throughout the sample and thus protons in different parts of the sample will resonate at slightly different frequencies. In addition, the protons will interact with each other causing a dephasing of their rotations about B_0 in a time characteristic of the system, called the spin–spin interaction time, T_2, and thus will precess at frequencies slightly different from ω_0.

In contrast to water, the proton NMR spectrum of ethyl alcohol (CH_3CH_2OH) exhibits some fine structure to the lineshape, because protons associated with each chemical group, i.e., CH_3, CH_2 and OH, experience slightly different electronic environments and thus the magnetic field (and consequently the resonant frequency) at each will be slightly different. This

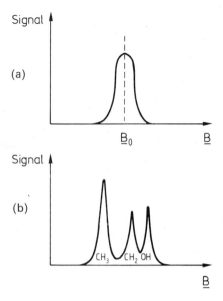

Figure 5. (a) Typical NMR absorption spectrum of water. (b) NMR absorption spectrum of ethyl alcohol.

phenomenon is known as chemical shift and a spectrum similar to that in figure 5(b) would be obtained. The three peaks are associated with the protons in each group. In both spectra in figure 5 the area under each peak is proportional to the number of protons in the sample.

To understand more fully the transitions involved within the spin system, and in particular the behaviour of the net magnetization M_0, it is instructive to introduce a rotating frame of coordinates where the frame rotates at the Larmor frequency. If the net magnetization is M_0 in the magnetic field direction after a system of protons has reached equilibrium within the field, then equation (1) can easily be generalised to

$$\frac{\mathrm{d}M_0}{\mathrm{d}t} = \gamma M_0 \wedge B_0 \tag{6}$$

If this equation is transposed to a frame rotating at frequency ω then we obtain

$$\left(\frac{\mathrm{d}M_0}{\mathrm{d}t}\right)_{\text{fixed frame}} = \left(\frac{\mathrm{d}M_0}{\mathrm{d}t}\right)_{\text{rotating frame}} + \omega \wedge M_0 \tag{7}$$

Substituting equation (6) in equation (7) and rearranging terms we obtain

$$\left(\frac{\mathrm{d}M_0}{\mathrm{d}t}\right)_{\text{rotating frame}} = \gamma M_0 \wedge (B_0 + \omega/\gamma) \tag{8}$$

where ω/γ has the dimensions of a magnetic field and is usually envisaged as a "fictitious" field arising from the rotation. We can now write

$$\left(\frac{\mathrm{d}M_0}{\mathrm{d}t}\right)_{\text{rotating frame}} = \gamma M_0 \wedge B_{\text{eff}} \tag{9}$$

where the effective field, $B_{\text{eff}} = B_0 + \omega/\gamma$; thus in the rotating frame M_0 precesses about B_{eff}. If we consider the case where B_0 only is present then $\omega = \omega_0 = -\gamma B_0$ (where the direction of ω_0 has been taken into account) and thus $B_{\text{eff}} = 0$. Under this condition M_0 is invariant in the rotating frame; this is just another statement of the Larmor precession condition described earlier. If an additional field B_1, rotating in the laboratory (fixed) frame at ω, is added to the system then

$$B_{\text{eff}} = B_0 + \omega/\gamma + B_1 \tag{10}$$

Now the resonance condition is $\omega = \omega_0 = -\gamma B_0$, i.e., the rotating frame has frequency of rotation ω_0, thus $B_{\text{eff}} = B_1$ and the magnetization M_0 rotates about B_1. If B_1 (rotating at $\omega = \omega_0$) is applied along the x'-axis (the x-axis

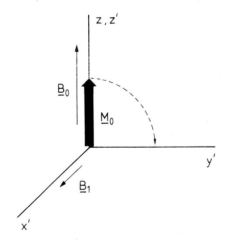

Figure 6. Precession of M_0 about B_1 in the rotating frame at resonance, i.e., $\omega = \omega_0 = -\gamma B_0$. The laboratory frame is given by x, y, z and the rotating frame x', y', z'.

in the rotating frame) then M_0 will rotate about the x'-axis (see figure 6). Equation (9) becomes

$$\left(\frac{\mathrm{d}M_0}{\mathrm{d}t}\right)_{\text{rotating frame}} = \gamma M_0 \wedge B_{\text{eff}} = \gamma M_0 \wedge B_1$$

and

$$|\omega_1| = \gamma |B_1| \tag{11}$$

where ω_1 = precessional frequency of M_0 about the x'-axis. This equation is similar to equations (3) and (4) where the Larmor frequency clearly depends on $|B_0|$. From equation (11) it can be seen that $|\omega_1|$ depends on $|B_1|$, which is usually of the order of 10^{-1}–10^{-2} T for most experiments, and for protons the precessional rate is approximately 10^6 rad s^{-1}. Thus if the radiofrequency radiation is applied for a short time, t_p (in seconds), then the angle θ through which M_0 precesses is given by

$$\theta = \gamma |B_1| t_p \tag{12}$$

This relationship is fundamental to the pulsed NMR technique. It is clear that if a burst of radiation is applied along x' (typically for 1 µs) then M_0 will tip towards the $x'y'$ plane (figure 6) and a component of M_0 will be generated along y'. A coil wrapped around a sample with its axis along the y-axis will have a small current induced in it, which can be detected by a system "tuned" to the Larmor frequency. In the laboratory frame of reference the motion of M_0 will be complex; however in the rotating frame M_0 will simply rotate about x'. Before the temporal development of M_0 can be considered further, relaxation mechanisms must be introduced.

1.4. Relaxation

After the net equilibrium magnetization M_0 has been disturbed by radio-frequency radiation at the Larmor frequency its return to alignment along B_0 is characterized by a time T_1, the spin–lattice relaxation time. This relaxation process involves the exchange of energy between the spin system (in our case this is essentially a free assembly of protons) and the lattice in which they are embedded, i.e., the molecular framework regardless of its physical state. In addition the spins can exchange energy amongst themselves giving rise to spin–spin relaxation with its characteristic time T_2. The return to equilibrium of the spin system via spin–lattice relaxation involves transitions of protons from the upper energy level to the lower (i.e., $n\downarrow$ to $n\uparrow$), whereas redistribution of energy amongst the spin system via spin–spin relaxation is accomplished by the transition of one proton from the higher to the lower energy level stimulating another proton to transfer from the lower to the higher level.

As mentioned previously it is usual to assign temperatures T_L and T_S to the lattice and spin systems respectively. In equilibrium $T_S = T_L = T$, where T is the temperature of the sample. The application of a pulse of radiofrequency radiation to a sample heats up the spin system causing T_S to change, because the population of the upper level increases and the lower decreases (equation (5)). After the radiation has been switched off the sample returns to equilibrium by cooling of the spin system. Thus T_S approaches T_L, which finally attains the bulk temperature of the sample T, because the lattice usually has a much higher thermal capacity than the spin system. The interactions within the spin and lattice systems are usually greater than that between the two systems, therefore it is reasonable to assign individual temperatures to each system.

1.4.1. Spin lattice relaxation

The approach to equilibrium of the spin and lattice systems after excitation by a burst of radiofrequency radiation is exponential and the rate of change of the magnetization M_z parallel to B_0 can be written

$$\frac{d|M_z|}{dt} = \frac{|M_0| - |M_z|}{T_1} \tag{13}$$

Typically T_1 ranges from 10^{-4} to 10^4 s and it is usually shorter in liquids than solids.

Spin–lattice relaxation is brought about by magnetic fields fluctuating at the correct frequency in the xy plane; they can then induce transitions between the upper and lower energy levels of the protons in the static magnetic field. If these fluctuations are associated with the lattice then exchange of energy between the spin and lattice systems can take place. In water this relaxation is brought about by the random motion of the water molecules (through their rotation and diffusion) causing the dipolar magnetic fields from the protons within them to fluctuate with time. Fluctuating fields from one proton at the Larmor frequency will be able to induce transitions between the upper and lower energy levels of neighbouring protons. This is the well known dipole–dipole interaction where the dipolar magnetic field falls off as r^{-3} where r is the distance between nearest neighbours.

The random motion of the molecules can be characterized by a correlation time τ_c which is usually found to follow a simple activation energy expression

$$\tau_c = \tau_0 \exp(E_A/kT_L) \tag{14}$$

where E_A is the activation energy, τ_0 the time constant characteristic of the motion, T_L the lattice temperature, and k is Boltzmann's constant.

For a randomly tumbling molecule the frequency distribution of the motion can be expressed as

$$J(\omega) = \frac{\tau_c}{1 + \omega^2 \tau_c{}^2} \tag{15}$$

where $J(\omega)$ is the spectral density function. Clearly T_1 will depend on $J(\omega)$ because fluctuating fields with a large spectral density at the Larmor frequency, ω_0, will excite transitions between the two levels. In addition T_1 will also depend on the magnitude of the magnetic fields in the xy plane $|B_{xy}|$, thus

$$\frac{1}{T_1} \propto |B_{xy}|^2 \frac{\tau_c}{1 + \omega^2 \tau_c{}^2} \tag{16}$$

It is easily seen from this equation that when $\tau_c = 1/\omega_0$, T_1 will go through a minimum because the mechanisms promoting relaxation will be most efficient when the molecules are reorienting at the Larmor frequency.

If a system such as water is considered in more detail it is found that an extra term involving transitions at 2ω must also be considered[5]. However the above arguments serve to illustrate the main features of the process.

The dipole–dipole interaction described above is one of six physical interactions that are generally important in the transfer of energy from the spin system to the lattice. The others are electric quadrupole, chemical shift anisotropy, indirect pseudo-dipolar, spin-rotation and paramagnetic centre interactions. In liquids the dipole–dipole interaction is dominant, in addition paramagnetic centres (when present), molecular oxygen for example, contribute to a shortening of T_1. Paramagnetic molecules are powerful in producing spin–lattice relaxation because their magnetic moments are essentially that of the electron, which is some 10^3 times greater than that of the nuclear magnetic moment, and so the fluctuating magnetic fields they produce are correspondingly stronger. Weak concentrations of paramagnetic materials will thus have a large effect on T_1 values.

1.4.2. Spin–spin relaxation

We have already seen that each proton produces a small magnetic field at its neighbour which falls off as r^{-3}, where r is the distance between neighbours. For water, each proton typically finds itself in a local field which ranges over $\pm 5 \times 10^{-4}$ T, hence the static field B_0 is spread over this range of values and the resonance condition is no longer sharp. A spread of resonance frequencies $\pm \Delta\omega_0$ will exist where $|\Delta\omega_0| = \gamma|\Delta B_0|$, thus the absorption line is broadened as in figure 5. For a system of protons $\Delta\omega_0 \sim 10^4$ s^{-1} and the individual protons lose phase with each other in times of the order of 10^{-4} s, simply because they precess at different frequencies. After the net magnetization (M_0) has been disturbed by a burst of radiofrequency radiation its components in the $x'y'$ plane will not remain constant in a particular direction but will decrease as the spins dephase.

A second dephasing process also occurs for identical nuclei whereby nucleus j can induce transitions of nucleus k by producing oscillating magnetic fields at its Larmor frequency. Thus a mutual exchange of energy can occur through spin exchange. This process produces further broadening of the absorption line.

It is convenient to introduce a spin–spin interaction time T_2 which describes the phase memory of the spin system and hence the decay of magnetization in a particular direction in the $x'y'$ plane after the equilibrium magnetization, M_0, has been tipped into this plane. The equations of motion are found to be

$$\frac{d|M_{x'}|}{dt} = -\frac{|M_{x'}|}{T_2}; \quad \frac{d|M_{y'}|}{dt} = -\frac{|M_{y'}|}{T_2} \tag{17}$$

In the rotating frame the component of the magnetization M_0 in the $x'y'$ plane will decay exponentially after it has been disturbed from its equilibrium configuration (i.e. $M_z = M_{z'} = M_0$ and $M_{x'} = M_{y'} = 0$).

Reorientation and diffusion of nuclei contribute to T_2 through the variations they produce, B_z and B_{xy} in B_0. The B_z variations are important for spin–spin interactions because it is variations in the precessional frequency of the nuclei that change their phase coherence. It should be noted that for spin–lattice interactions it is only varying fields perpendicular to B_0, i.e., B_{xy}, that are important because these can induce transitions between the two energy levels.

For liquids and gases local magnetic field variations are smoothed out since the reorientation and diffusion of molecules within the system are rapid, thus the absorption lines are narrow because local field variations are averaged nearly to zero. In solids, however, broader absorption lines are observed because these variations are not averaged.

There are two other additional forms of broadening of the absorption line. The first is inhomogeneities in the static field B_0, which act like local field contributions to B_0 from other nuclei. It is found that

$$\frac{1}{T_2{}^*} = \frac{1}{T_2} + \frac{\gamma |\Delta B_0|}{2} \tag{18}$$

where $T_2{}^*$ is the observed spin–spin relaxation time, which includes contributions from both natural linewidth processes and magnetic field inhomogeneities. T_2 is the actual spin–spin relaxation time and ΔB_0 is the variation in the static magnetic field over the sample. The absorption curve linewidth $\Delta \omega_0$ is given by $1/T_2{}^* = \Delta \omega_0/2$. The second additional broadening mechanism arises if T_1 is very short and thus the lifetime of a given nucleus in a particular state is brief. This will lead to lifetime broadening where the uncertainty in the resonant frequency $\Delta \omega_0 \sim 1/T_1$.

In general, therefore, after the spin system has been disturbed the magnetization in the $x'y'$ plane in a particular direction tends to zero, with no exchange of energy with the lattice, in a characteristic time T_2. In addition, the spin system will also exchange energy with the lattice so that the equilibrium magnetization M_0 is again established with a characteristic time T_1 which is greater than T_2; the latter condition usually pertains in liquids. From the foregoing remarks it can be seen that all processes that contribute to spin–lattice relaxation will also produce spin–spin relaxation and thus T_2 will always be less than T_1.

Measurements of T_1 and T_2 lead to information about molecular structure and mobility. The spin–spin interaction time can give information about diffusion rates, for example, diffusion of molecules across membranes. Spin–lattice relaxation time has been found to vary markedly from one type of tissue to another (see, for example, Gore[6], Ling et al.[7]) and for this reason T_1 is mapped to produce contrast in NMR imaging.

1.5. Pulsed NMR experiment

Consider a system of protons (such as a water sample) immersed in a static field B_0 so that M_0 is directed along the z-axis in the laboratory reference frame. If a pulse of radiofrequency radiation at the Larmor frequency (ω_0) is applied along x' (x-axis in the rotating frame) for a time t_p (equation (12)) so that M_0 is tipped into the $x'y'$ plane, the burst of radiofrequency radiation is called a 90° pulse (figure 7(a, b)).

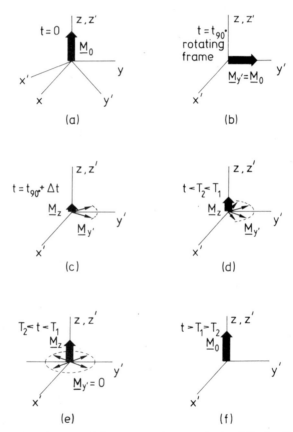

Figure 7. Temporal development of the macroscopic magnetization following the application of a 90° pulse.

The temporal development of magnetization in the xy plane can be measured using a detector coil wound round the sample and aligned along the y-axis and tuned to ω_0 (thus it effectively monitors signals along the y'-axis). In this way the magnetization along the y'-axis ($M_{y'}$) can be monitored by measuring the currents induced in the detector coil. After M_0 has been turned into the $x'y'$ plane the protons contributing to the net magnetization can effectively be thought of as a separate system. These protons then interact amongst themselves (spin–spin interactions) and cause a spread of precessional frequencies about the z-axis so that in a short time the proton spins fan out in the $x'y'$ plane and $M_{y'}$ decays with time constant T_2^* (equation (18), figure 7(c)).

This decay of $M_{y'}$ induces a changing current in the detector coil (the maximum being proportional to M_0) which falls to zero as $M_{y'}$ decays from $|M_0|$ to zero. An exponential decay is usually observed for liquids (equation (17)) and is called the free induction decay (FID), the time constant of which is T_2^*. Typically, the signal from the receiver coil is amplified and then displayed on an oscilloscope (figure 8). If the detector system is not tuned

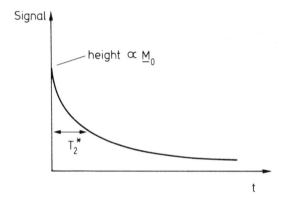

Figure 8. Free induction decay (FID) following a 90° pulse.

to ω_0 then a decaying oscillating signal would be observed, the envelope of which is the FID. Fourier transformation of the FID following a 90° pulse of radiofrequency radiation gives the NMR absorption spectrum (Lowe and Norberg[8]).

At the same time as the spins dephase they relax back to their equilibrium configuration (i.e., M_0 aligned along B_0) by giving up energy to the lattice (spin–lattice relaxation). In this way magnetization in the xy plane gradually decreases to zero (figure 7(c)–(f)). In contrast, a 180° pulse would turn the magnetization into the negative z-direction and thus no signal would be measured along y'.

In summary, therefore, immediately after a 90° pulse M_z changes rapidly from M_0 to zero and $M_{y'}$ increases from zero to M_0. After further time $M_{y'}$ decays to zero with characteristic time T_2 and M_z gradually returns to M_0 with time constant T_1.

1.6. Measurements of T_1 and T_2

Both T_1 and T_2 can be measured by the application of suitable sequences of
90° and 180° pulses to a sample. Some of the more common systems are
outlined below.

1.6.1. T_1 measurements

(i) $90° - \tau - 90°$ sequence

In this system a 90° pulse is applied to the sample and then after a time τ
(less than T_1) a further 90° inspection pulse is applied to determine how much
of the equilibrium magnetization ($|M_0|$) has relaxed back to the z-direction.
The maximum height of the FID, $A(\tau)$, after the second pulse is smaller than
that after the first because only a fraction of the spins will have relaxed back
to precessing about the field B_0 (figure 9). It should be noted that a 90° pulse
gives a measure of the net magnetization in the z-direction at any time.

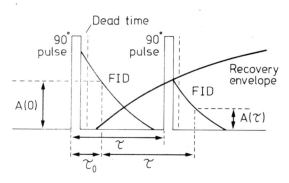

Figure 9. $90° - \tau - 90°$ pulse sequence for measuring T_1. The recovery envelope of the amplitude
of the FID, $A(\tau)$, as a function of τ is indicated.

After the spin system has been allowed to return to equilibrium with the
lattice (a time of approximately $5T_1$) another sequence of two 90° pulses is
applied to the system with a different spacing τ between the pulses. Again
the recovery of the magnetization in the z-direction can be found by
monitoring the height of the second FID. Further sequences enable the whole
of the function $A(\tau)$ to be measured. Usually the detecting system has an
inherent "dead-time" and thus a point τ_0 after the beginning of the FID is
chosen to measure $A(\tau)$, the height of the FID after each $90° - \tau - 90°$
sequence (figure 9). The amplitude $A(0)$ of the FID after a single 90° pulse
gives a measure of M_0. It is readily seen that $M_z \propto A(\tau)$, and thus from
equation (13) it is clear that

$$A(\tau) = A(0)[1 - \exp(-\tau/T_1)] \tag{20}$$

By plotting $\ln[A(0) - A(\tau)]$ against τ a straight line is obtained, the slope of which gives T_1.

Deviation from linearity of the plot of $\ln[A(0) - A(\tau)]$ against τ indicates that a non-exponential recovery of the magnetization is present, due to protons contributing to the NMR signal from different physical states. This may be the case for the behaviour of protons in human tissue where they find themselves in many different environments, for example, bound to cell constituents, or essentially free, as water in extracellular fluid.

(ii) $180° - \tau - 90°$ sequence (inversion recovery)

For this sequence a $180°$ pulse is used to invert the equilibrium magnetization M_0 along z to the $-z$-direction, i.e., $M_z = -M_0$. Spin–lattice relaxation then takes place and the magnetization along z is gradually restored to M_0. Application of a $90°$ pulse a time τ after the $180°$ pulse will then tip any magnetization along z into the $x'y'$ plane, which will induce a signal in the receiver coil, the amplitude of which is given by

$$A(\tau) = A(0)\left[1 - 2\exp\left(-\frac{\tau}{T_1} \right) \right] \tag{21}$$

As with the $90° - \tau - 90°$ sequence a value for T_1 can be found by determining the value of $A(\tau)$ for different τ. This sequence is illustrated in figure (10) where it should be noted that at $\tau = T_1 \ln 2$, $A(\tau) = 0$, and thus T_1 can be found in principle from a single measurement of the τ value required to produce a null signal when the $90°$ pulse is applied. In practice, however, an

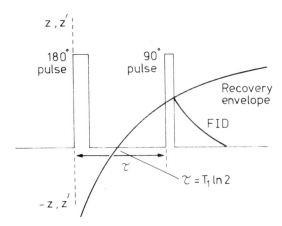

Figure 10. $180 - \tau - 90$ pulse sequence for measuring T_1. The recovery envelope of the amplitude of the FID, $A(\tau)$, is indicated. The initial 180 inverts the equilibrium magnetization M_0 to the $-z$-direction.

exponential fit is done to the values obtained for several different τ or, in imaging, equation (21) is solved for perhaps two τ values.

1.6.2. T_2 measurements

(i) Spin–echo sequence

Although this sequence does not yield the most accurate determination of T_2 it is described here as it is the basis of T_2 measurements in other pulse sequences.

It can be seen from equation (18) that magnetic field inhomogeneities contribute to T_2, and unless $T_2 \ll 2/\gamma|\Delta B_0|$ they preclude the measurement of T_2 directly from the FID; only T_2^* can be measured. A $90° - \tau - 180°$ sequence can be used [9,10] to overcome these difficulties in which a $90°$ pulse is first applied to the sample and then a time τ later a $180°$ pulse inverts the magnetization in the $x'y'$ plane and subsequently, at a further time τ, a spin–echo signal is observed. The method is best understood by considering figure 11. After the $90°$ pulse (along x') the magnetization M_0 is turned into the $x'y'$ plane along y', i.e., the individual protons precess about z in the x, y plane of the laboratory (figure 11(a)). The protons then dephase relative to each other due to magnetic field inhomogeneities and spin–spin relaxation— some precess faster than ω_0 and some slower (figure 11(b)). If a $180°$ pulse is applied along x' a time τ after the $90°$ pulse the protons will now be rotated $180°$ about x' and those that were rotating clockwise in the $x'y'$ plane (due to the spread of ω_0) will rotate counterclockwise and vice versa (note that this motion is now all referred to the rotating frame) (figure 11(c)). Clearly a further time τ after the $180°$ pulse the individual protons will cross the $-y'$-axis together and a negative signal will build up and decay in the receiver coil (figure 11(e) and (g)), after which the protons will continue to dephase (figure 11(f)). In this way the amplitude of the spin–echo signal will be governed by T_2 and τ because spin–spin relaxation will have taken place and the effects of magnetic field inhomogeneities are essentially eliminated if the individual protons remain in the same magnetic field throughout the experiment, that is, the inverting $180°$ pulse cancels out any static magnetic field inhomogeneity effects. If molecular diffusion takes place between the $90°$ and $180°$ pulses then the echo amplitude will be affected by the different magnetic fields experienced by individual protons as they move and the amplitude of the echo signal a time 2τ after the $90°$ pulse is given by:

$$A(2\tau) = A(0)\exp\left(-\frac{2\tau}{T_2} - \frac{2}{3}\gamma^2 G^2 D\tau^3 \right) \tag{22}$$

where G is the spatial magnetic field gradient, and D is the diffusion coefficient.

Clearly the second term in the exponent of this expression becomes more pronounced for longer τ values (due to the τ^3 dependence) and therefore this

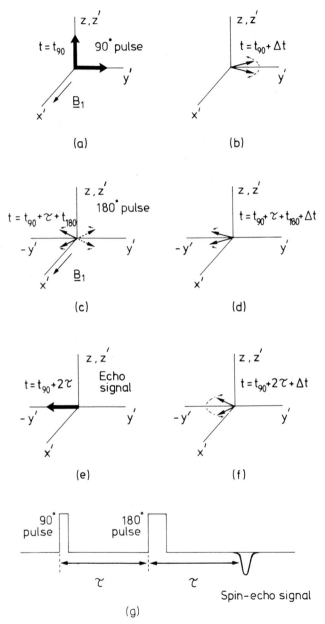

Figure 11. $90° - \tau - 180°$ pulse sequence for measuring T_2, spin–echo. The motion of the individual protons in the $x'y'$ plane is indicated schematically. In addition the formation of the echo signal is shown.

method is only applicable for short T_2 values. Measurement of $A(2\tau)$ as a function of τ will yield a value of T_2 as long as diffusion effects are small. As with T_1 measurements, a time approximately $5T_1$ must elapse between each sequence to allow the sample to reach equilibrium.

(ii) Carr–Purcell sequence

To overcome the problems of diffusion Carr and Purcell[11] suggested a modification to the spin–echo technique in which a train of 180° pulses are applied after the first 90° pulse, i.e., a sequence of $90° - \tau - 180° - 2\tau - 180° - 2\tau \ldots$ etc. (the Carr–Purcell sequence) and with all the pulses applied along the x'-axis. The process proceeds as in figure 11(a)–(f) but after the echo signal and further dephasing of the protons another 180° pulse is applied a time 3τ after the first 90° pulse, which produces a second echo in the $+y'$ direction at a time 4τ. Subsequent 180° pulses at times 5τ, $7\tau \ldots$ etc. are then applied which will produce alternative positive and negative echoes at 6τ, $8\tau \ldots$ etc.

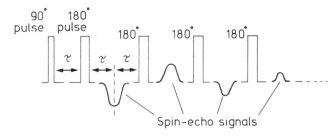

Figure 12. Carr–Purcell sequence showing the formation of echo signals at times 2τ, $4\tau \ldots$ etc. after the 90° pulse.

(figure 12). The amplitude of these echoes is given by:

$$A(t) = A(0)\exp\left[-\frac{t}{T_2} - \frac{1}{3}\gamma^2 G^2 D\tau^2 t \right] \tag{23}$$

where t is the length of time over which the pulse sequence is applied, usually long compared with τ. During each time τ after the 180° pulse, spin–spin relaxation takes place and the amplitude of each echo will be reduced. It is possible, therefore, to reduce considerably the effect of diffusion by choosing a short τ, thereby making the second term in equation (23) negligible. The envelope of the echo amplitudes (figure 12) is then governed by T_2. This method not only overcomes problems with diffusion but also makes the measuring time short, only one sequence lasting approximately for T_2 is required, whereas for the spin–echo method a number of $90° - \tau - 180°$ pulse sequences are required with a time $5T_1$ between each sequence. For measurements of long T_2, however, a large number of 180° pulses are required and inaccuracies will occur if the 180° pulse lengths and B_1 are not constant. This can be overcome by a modification to this technique proposed by Meiboom and Gill[12]—the Carr–Purcell Meiboon–Gill sequence (CPMG) in which the same basic pulse sequence utilized in the Carr–Purcell technique is used; the 180° pulses, however, are applied along the y'-axis, i.e., $\pi/2$ out of phase with the initial 90° pulse.

References

1. Bloch F, Hanson W W and Packard M 1946 *Physical Review* **70** 474
2. Bloch F 1946 *Physical Review* **70** 460
3. Abragam A 1960 *The Principles of Nuclear Magnetism* (Oxford University Press)
4. Slichter C P 1964 *Magnetic Resonance* (New York: Harper and Row)
5. Andrew E R 1969 *Nuclear Magnetic Resonance* (Cambridge University Press)
6. Gore J C 1981, in *Proceedings of an International Symposium on Nuclear Magnetic Resonance Imaging, Wake Forest University, USA* (Bowman Gray School of Medicine Press)
7. Ling C R, Foster M A and Hutchison J M S 1980 *Physics in Medicine and Biology* **25** 748
8. Lowe I S and Norberg R E 1957 *Physical Review* **107** 46
9. Hahn H L 1950 *Physical Review* **80** 580
10. Farrar T C and Becker E D 1971 *Pulse and Fourier Transform NMR* (New York: Academic Press)
11. Carr H Y and Purcell E M 1954 *Physical Review* **94** 630
12. Meiboom S and Gill D 1958 *Review of Scientific Instruments* **29** 688

D G Taylor and R Inamdar

Department of Physics, University of Surrey,
Guildford GU2 5XH, England

2.1. Introduction

In this chapter, we describe the design, logic, and operation of a typical NMR imaging system. The aim is to provide the reader with an understanding of NMR imaging instrumentation and to indicate the features common to most systems.

To produce an image, the sample is subjected to a strong, uniform magnetic field. Gradient coils modulate this uniform field in a manner determined by the imaging technique in use. Resonance is induced by radiofrequency (RF) radiation delivered from a transmitter through an antenna or probe. The same or a second probe detects the resulting NMR signals, which are suitably amplified and filtered before digitization and input to a computer system. In addition, the computer system provides the functions of control, data processing, and display.

The imaging system can be divided into a number of units; (1) the magnet, (2) the transmitter, (3) the probe, (4) the gradient system, (5) the receiver, and (6) the computer system. In this chapter we discuss in some detail each of these units except for the magnet, which is described elsewhere. However, before discussing the instrumentation it is helpful to consider practical methods of inducing resonance.

2.1.1. Pulsed NMR

In NMR imaging, information is contained in the amplitude and phase of an absorption spectrum. In conventional spectroscopy, to determine that spectrum one would sweep the frequency of the incident radiation. However, in NMR it is possible to excite the whole spectrum using pulsed radiation techniques. The pulse must be of sufficiently short duration to contain a uniform spread of frequencies over the bandwidth to be excited. The frequency content of any RF pulse may be determined by a simple Fourier transform[1]. For example, for a rectangular RF pulse, $p(t)$

$$p(t) = A \cos(\omega_0 t + \phi) \cdot e(t)$$

where the envelope $e(t) = 0$ for $t < 0$ and $t > t_p$

and $\qquad = 1$ for $0 \leqslant t \leqslant t_p$

Fourier transforming, we obtain

$$P(\omega) = \int\limits_{-\infty}^{+\infty} p(t)e^{i\omega t}\mathrm{d}t$$

$$= \delta(\omega - \omega_0) \otimes \cdot E(\omega)$$

that is, a delta function at the resonant frequency ω_0 convoluted with the Fourier transform of the pulse envelope, which in this case is given by

$$E(\omega) = \frac{\sin(\omega t)}{\omega t}$$

as shown in figure 1.

Since it is not possible to collimate RF radiation, techniques are required to restrict the irradiation to a limited region, for example, a thin cross-section.

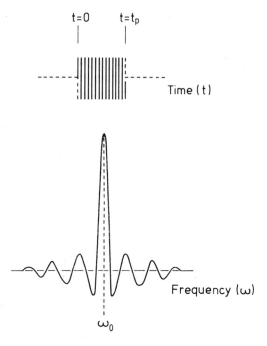

Figure 1. The Fourier transform of a rectangular radiofrequency pulse.

2.1.2. Selective irradiation

Consider an extended cylindrical sample. We wish to irradiate a thin cross-sectional region transverse to the longitudinal direction. If we apply a linear magnetic field gradient in the longitudinal direction, the absorption frequency is a function of position in this direction. Irradiation with a pulse containing a very narrow rectangular envelope of frequencies will then only excite the desired cross-section as shown in the diagram (figure 2).

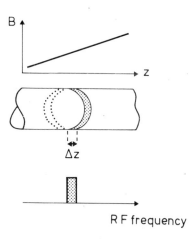

Figure 2. Selective irradiation of a slice in a sample in the presence of a gradient in the z direction.

Following irradiation, gradients in the x and y directions are applied to encode spatial information within this cross-section.

It is readily seen from the analysis given in the previous section that to produce a rectangular envelope of frequencies a sinc shaped envelope must be generated in the time domain. However a sinc function extends to infinity, and in the practical implementation it must be truncated. As a consequence distortions in the form of ripples arise in the frequency envelope. To minimize these distortions the pulse envelope in the time domain is weighted with a damping function, typically a Gaussian, Ce^{-dt^2}. The resulting frequency envelope is shown in figure 3.

We must now consider the response of the nuclei within the slice to this irradiation sequence. The equation of motion in the rotating frame of the nuclear magnetization, M_0 is given by

$$\frac{\mathrm{d}M_0}{\mathrm{d}t} = \gamma M_0 \wedge B_{\text{eff}}$$

where $B_{\text{eff}} = B_1(z) + G_z z$

In the absence of the gradient and sufficiently intense B_1, the nuclear

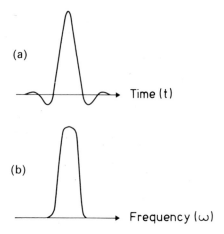

Figure 3. (a) The weighting of a truncated sinc function with a Gaussian, in the time domain, and (b) its Fourier transform in the frequency domain.

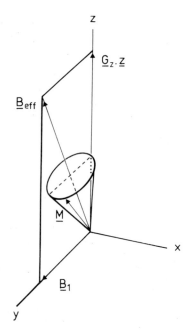

Figure 4. Sketch showing the motion of the magnetization M, in the rotating frame, in the presence of a radiofrequency field B_1 and a longitudinal field gradient G_z.

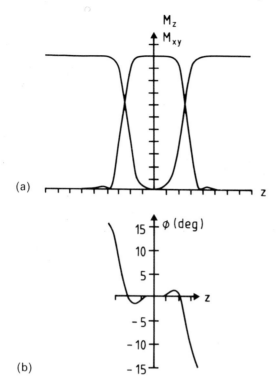

Figure 5. (a) Magnetization at the end of a selective 90° radiofrequency pulse. (b) The residual phase error at the centre of the echo following gradient reversal.

moments would precess coherently about B_{eff}. However, due to the presence of the gradient, nuclei at each position along the longitudinal direction will experience a different B_{eff} (see figure 4). This results in a rapid loss of phase coherence of the nuclear moments such that at the end of, for example, a 90° pulse, they are widely distributed in the xy plane of the rotating frame.

The response of any position within the selected cross-section may be computed numerically by integration of the equation of motion given above. It can be shown for a 90° pulse that the variation of phase with z is approximately linear. This permits phase coherence to be recovered by a simple longitudinal gradient reversal for a length of time approximately half that of the irradiating pulse (figure 5).

This subject has been treated by several authors (Hoult[2], Sutherland and Hutchison[3], and Mansfield *et al.*[4]) For a detailed analysis readers are referred to the book by Mansfield and Morris[5].

For pulse angles much greater than 90° a simple gradient reversal is no longer adequate to restore coherence. The generation of a satisfactory selective 180° pulse is still under investigation by a number of groups.

Summarizing, selective irradiation requires application of a linear magnetic field gradient, irradiation with a modulated radiofrequency pulse, and finally a gradient reversal for a period of time usually determined experimentally.

2.2. The imaging system

There are two basic methods of encoding spatial information, frequency and phase encoding: however, within these two broad categories a multitude of variants have been developed. A typical pulse sequence is shown in figure 6.

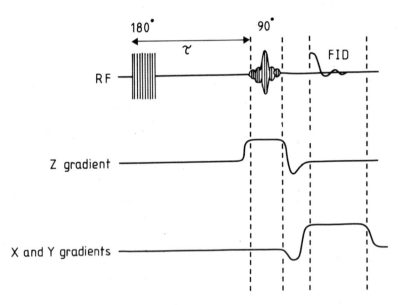

Figure 6. An example of an inversion recovery imaging pulse sequence utilizing back projection reconstruction.

The diagram is for an inversion recovery sequence, $180° - \tau - 90°$. The 180° pulse is non-selective, unlike the 90° pulse which is used to define the required cross-section. Information within the image plane is encoded in frequency by the X and Y gradients. The final image is reconstructed from projections.

A well designed NMR imaging system should be capable of implementing any of the possible imaging methods with changes required only in the software for computer control and data processing. A schematic diagram of a complete system is shown in figure 7.

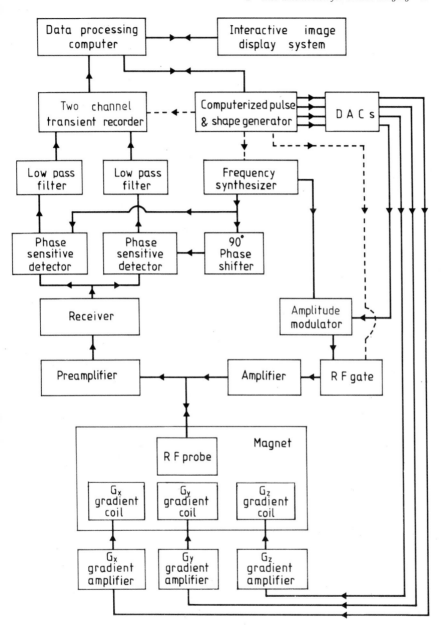

Figure 7. Schematic diagram of an NMR imaging system.

It is convenient to separate the functions of data processing and control. A dedicated microprocessor is normally used for control and a larger computer system for data collection, processing and display. Thus in normal operation, on command from the main computer system, the microprocessor sets the X, Y and Z gradients to appropriate values at the appropriate time via three digital to analogue convertors (DACs) followed by amplification stages.

Similarly, modulated RF pulses are generated using a fourth DAC and modulator. The pulses are then fed to the probe within the magnet and the resulting NMR signal is detected by a receiver system. Finally the signals are digitized and input to the main computer for processing.

2.3. The transmitter

The function of the transmitter is to irradiate the sample with RF fields of the appropriate frequency content, power and timing. The transmitter system consists of a frequency synthesizer, and amplitude modulator, a "gate" which

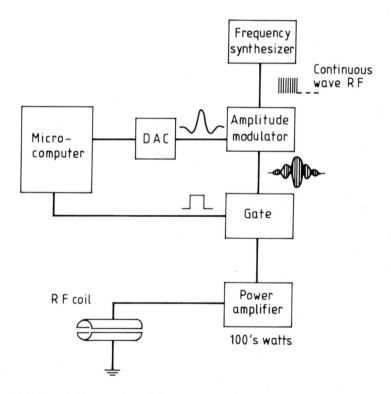

Figure 8. Schematic diagram of a radiofrequency transmitter.

switches the transmission on and off at the required times, and a power amplifier which boosts the RF power to the appropriate level (see figure 8).

A standard crystal oscillator operating at a fixed frequency with thermal control may be used as the frequency generator. This device is capable of producing a frequency with an accuracy of $1:10^7$ or better. However, for flexibility it is more common to use a variable frequency synthesizer, preferably one that may be controlled from the computer system, permitting a rapid change in frequency and phase of the irradiating signal. The output from the synthesizer has a power level of about 2 V peak-to-peak into a 50 Ω load. The whole system is normally matched to 50 Ω as 50 Ω matched components are widely available, enabling the rapid construction of the RF system as a set of plug-in modules.

As we have seen, the technique of selective irradiation requires amplitude modulation of the radiofrequency signal. There are a number of devices which will provide this function; the authors, for example, use a Hatfield Instruments double balanced Mixer Type 1754. The modulating signal is provided by a DAC under computer control. The modulating function, having been previously determined analytically, is normally stored in the form of a look-up table in the computer memory or a buffer memory. The modulation circuit in general has inadequate isolation in its OFF state. Any leakage of RF will be amplified by the transmitter amplifier, fed to the probe and detected by the very sensitive receiving circuitry. An isolation of 120 dB or better is required: this is provided by the radiofrequency gate. The control system must therefore open this gate simultaneously with the output of the modulating function.

Finally the RF pulse is fed to an amplifier before transmission to the probe. The RF power required depends very much on the imaging method used and also on the transmitter coil design and tuning arrangement. The power requirements for selective irradiation are very low, typically a few watts for a 90° pulse of duration ~ 5 ms. For non-selective techniques, especially driven equilibrium methods, much higher powers are required, typically 4 to 5 kW for 10 µs 90° pulses. Although the bandwidth required even for the shortest pulse is quite small, ~ 100 kHz maximum, it is easier to use a commercial broad-band amplifier of the requisite power and frequency range and not tune the system until the probe.

2.4. The probe

The design of the radiofrequency probe is of paramount importance in the study of biological systems. The quality of the probe design very largely determines the performance of an imaging system. The probe is essentially an antenna, that is, a coil around the patient. Sometimes the same coil is used to irradiate and detect the NMR signal or a different coil may be used for detection. The design aim in both receiver and transmitter coils is to produce uniform magnetic fields over as large a fraction of the coil volume as possible. Further, it is essential to optimize the signal-to-noise ratio (SNR) if we wish to obtain acceptable images in a minimum time.

Conventional radiofrequency coils are usually either solenoidal or saddle-shaped (see figure 9). Almost all imaging magnets have the field B_0 directed along the longitudinal axis of the patient, and therefore the radiofrequency field B_1 must be applied in the transverse plane. A saddle-shaped coil can

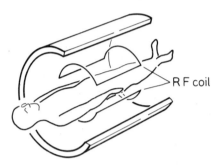

Figure 9. Sketch showing the position of the radiofrequency coil with respect to the magnet and patient.

be oriented as shown in figure 9, which permits easy access for the patient: however, it is not possible to use solenoidal coils, unless the B_0 field is transverse to the patient, due to the problem of access. An outline will be given of the design considerations for optimum RF homogeneity and signal-to-noise ratio. For more extensive discussions, the reader is referred to the books of Mansfield and Morris[5] and Gadian[6].

2.4.1. Coil design

The total magnetic field produced at the point P distant r from a current I flowing in a wire is given by the Biot-Savart expression:

$$B = \frac{\mu_0 I}{4\pi} \int \frac{dl \times \hat{r}}{r^2}$$

where $\hat{r}$ is the unit vector between the conductor line element dl at the point P, and μ_0 is the permeability of free space.

This equation may be simply integrated to obtain the field at point P for any given wire configuration. For example, the field at a point distant r from the middle of a straight wire of length $2l$ along the z-axis is

$$B = \frac{\mu_0 I}{2\pi r} \frac{l}{(l^2 + r^2)^{\frac{1}{2}}}$$

This is a field tangential to a circle coaxial with z. In the limit $l \to \infty$ we obtain the well known result

$$B = \frac{\mu_0 I}{2\pi r}$$

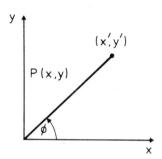

Figure 10. The coordinates and axes of a conductor at (x', y') and the point (x, y).

Consider this wire displaced from the origin to coordinates (x', y') in the x, y plane (figure 10). The component of the field at point $P(x, y)$ along the x direction is given by

$$B_x(x, y) = \frac{\mu_0 I}{2\pi} \frac{(y' - y)}{(x' - x)^2 + (y' - y)^2}$$

Following Zupančič and Pirš[7] this can be written as the real part of the complex function

$$B_x(x, y) = \frac{\mu_0 I}{2\pi} \text{Re}\{[(y' + ix') - (y + ix)]^{-1}\}$$

Let

$$(y + ix) = \alpha$$

and

$$(y' + ix') = re^{i\phi}$$

then the above equation may be expanded as a Taylor series provided $|\alpha| < r$. In this case we may write

$$B_x(x, y) = \frac{\mu_0 I}{2\pi r} \text{Re} \sum_{n=0}^{\infty} \left(\frac{\alpha}{r}\right)^n \exp[-i(n + 1)\phi]$$

This expansion converges rapidly and is useful for estimating the main field contributions for a particular set of straight conductors and current directions. For example, the optimum geometry may be determined for a four-wire coil

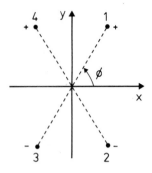

Figure 11. The positions of four infinite wires and the current directions that will produce a uniform field B_1 along x, provided $\phi = 60°$.

with wires arranged as in figure 11. From the symmetry of the conductors, the fields produced by wire pairs 1, 3 and 2, 4 contain only even orders of the parameter α/r. Summing all components we obtain

$$B_x = \frac{2\mu_0 I}{\pi r} \text{Re}\left[1 - i(\alpha/r)^2 \sin 3\phi - i(\alpha/r)^4 \sin 5\phi + \ldots\right]$$

If $\phi = 60°$ the third order term vanishes and the field to the third order is given by $B = 2\mu_0 I / \pi r$.

Most non-solenoidal coil system designs are based on the field produced by four wires in the configuration above. In the practical situation, these wires cannot of course be infinitely long, and designs differ predominantly in the layout of the return paths. The simplest configuration is that shown in figure 12 where the return paths are straight, forming a rectangular coil

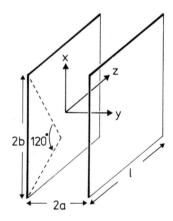

Figure 12. A rectangular coil pair of length l and spacing $2a$. The field is produced along the y-axis.

pair. Mansfield and Morris[5] have shown that this configuration produces excellent field uniformity (to better than 5%) over most of the useable cross-section of the mid-xy plane when $l/b = 2$. Further, this configuration produces high RF field per unit current, approximately twice that of the saddle-shape arrangement shown in figure 9. In addition, the homogeneity of the saddle arrangement is only good to 10% for the typical configuration of length:radius ratio = 2. The saddle arrangement does, however, have the very strong advantage of permitting maximum access. Thus in the restricted environment of a whole-body magnet most designers have opted for this configuration.

Finally, one further important consideration must be taken into account when designing a coil system. If the total length of wire used becomes significant compared with the wavelength of the radiation, then serious phase shifts may be incurred by the RF signal as it passes down the length of the coil. This will result in substantial inhomogeneities in the RF field. Hoult[8] has therefore suggested that, as a rule of thumb, the total length of wire should not exceed $\lambda/20$.

2.4.2. Signal-to-noise considerations

Consider a solenoidal coil surrounding a sample and suppose a 90° pulse has just been applied. The magnetization which precesses with angular frequency ω_0 induces an EMF of the same frequency in the coil. The magnitude ε of the EMF is given by Faraday's law,

$$\varepsilon = -\frac{d\phi}{dt}$$

where ϕ is the magnetic flux linkage through the coil. The EMF constitutes the NMR signal. Hoult and Richards[9] calculated the total EMF produced by a sample of volume V, situated in a region of homogeneous B_1 field, following a 90° pulse as

$$\varepsilon = \omega_0 B_{1u} M_0 V$$

where B_{1u} is the field generated in the xy plane by unit current passing through the coil. The nuclear magnetization M_0 is given by

$$M_0 = N\gamma^2\hbar^2 I(I + 1)(B_0/3kT)$$

where N is number of resonant nuclei per unit volume, γ is the gyromagnetic ratio of these nuclei, T is the sample temperature, and k is the Boltzmann constant: thus the signal generated in the coil may be evaluated.

To determine the signal-to-noise ratio (SNR) an estimate of the noise that is generated in the experiment must be made. In a well designed system almost all the noise originates in the radiofrequency coil (ignoring for the moment, the noise generated by the sample). The noise developed in the coil is that due to thermal motion of the electrons. The root mean square of the EMF over a bandwidth Δv at ω_0 is given by

$$n = (4kT_cR_c\Delta v)^{\frac{1}{2}}$$

where R_c is the resistance of the coil and T_c its temperature. To optimize the signal-to-noise we wish to maximize the ratio ε/n, which at a fixed frequency and temperature reduces to maximizing $NV \cdot B_{1u}/R_c^{\frac{1}{2}}$. It should be noted that the parameters B_{1u}, R_c and V are not independent variables, as they are dependent on the dimensions of the coil.

Solenoidal coils produce greater SNR than saddle-shaped coils for a given sample volume. The ratio $B_{1u}/R_c^{\frac{1}{2}}$ is greater for a solenoid than for a saddle-shaped coil. A saddle-shaped coil requires a longer length of wire to generate a given B_1 field and hence has a greater resistance than a solenoidal coil. In general, for optimally designed coils, sensitivity of the solenoidal coil is expected to be better by a factor of 2.

Living systems have a fairly high concentration of ions and, as a result, conduct electricity. This can have profound consequences as the sample itself can generate a significant amount of noise, thus decreasing the effective SNR. In addition there will be a limitation on the depth of penetration of the RF field into the sample. There are two major loss mechanisms, magnetic losses and dielectric losses.

Magnetic losses arise due to the back EMF induced in the sample itself following the induction of the EMF in the receiving coil. If the sample is conducting, currents flow within it and these "eddy" currents dissipate power. This power loss is equivalent to the power losses within the resistance of the coil itself and represents an additional source of resistance R_m. The total effective resistance R_T can now be written $R_T = R_c + R_m$ and the SNR is therefore proportional to $B_{1u}V/(R_c + R_m)^{\frac{1}{2}}$. Hoult and Lauterbur[10] have shown that for a cylindrical sample enclosed by a solenoidal coil, $R_m = V^2B_{1u}^2\omega_0^2\rho/16\pi g$, where ρ is the conductivity of the sample and $2g$ is the length of both sample and coil. It should be noted that if the condition $R_m > R_c$ is reached any improvement in the coil design will have very little effect on the SNR: therefore to optimize SNR we should attempt to approach this limiting condition.

Dielectric losses arise when electric fields produce electric lines of force which pass through a conducting sample. Just as with magnetic losses, this can be represented by an effective resistance R_e. Attempts have been made to screen these electric fields from entering the sample but with limited success. In practice, coils can be designed such that dielectric losses are small compared with magnetic losses and coil losses.

Summarizing, the objective is to design a radiofrequency probe that produces maximum B_1 homogeneity over the sample volume and maximum RF field per unit current for the minimum length of coil conductor. The resistance of the coil at the resonant frequency should be minimized by the use of a high purity annealed copper conductor having a large surface area to allow for the skin-depth effect. In addition, the layout should attempt to minimize stray capacitance and all lead lengths should be kept to a minimum. Finally the tuned circuit, of which the probe forms a part, should be impedance matched to the transmitter for maximum power transfer, and optimum noise matched to the receiver for maximum signal-to-noise ratio. These are often conflicting requirements and may be overcome by the use of a cross-coil system. A tuned circuit commonly used in NMR probes is shown in figure 13.

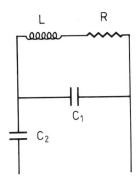

Figure 13. A tuned circuit for a single coil probe.

The use of two tuning capacitors C_1 and C_2 permits both the resonant frequency and the impedance of the circuit to be set independently. A full analysis of this circuit is given by Hoult[11].

2.5. The gradient system

The objective of the gradient coil system is to produce gradients $G_z = \partial B_z/\partial z$, $G_x = \partial B_z/\partial x$ and $G_y = \partial B_z/\partial y$. As with radiofrequency coils, there are a number of conductor configurations that may be used. A widely adopted configuration is shown in figure 14. A pair of circular coils of radius a in a Helmholtz configuration but with opposing currents are used to generate G_z. The optimum field gradient linearity is obtained when the coils are spaced $a\sqrt{3}$ apart. Each of the G_x and G_y gradients is produced by a pair of saddle coils. The direction of current flow between the members of a pair is reversed. The G_x and G_y gradient coils are identical but rotated through $90°$ about the longitudinal axis with respect to each other.

In general it is not possible or desirable to switch these gradients sharply on and off due to the intrinsic inductance of the coils and the eddy currents induced in the body of the magnet system. The gradients are normally driven by digital to analogue convertors through current amplifiers under computer control. This permits a controlled switch on and switch off as well as accurate

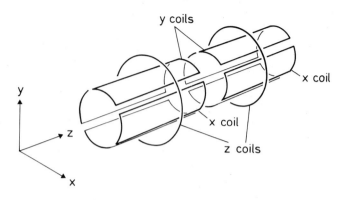

Figure 14. Sketch showing the position of the field gradient coils.

control of the final gradient strength. For accuracy, 12 bit DACs are used giving a 1:4096 amplitude resolution. The Amcron M600 is used by most commercial organizations as the gradient amplifier and produces approximately 20 A at 80 V. The ultimate gradient strength required depends on many factors such as magnet homogeneity and imaging technique, but gradient strengths are typically of the order 0.5 mT m^{-1}.

2.6. The receiver system

A schematic diagram of the receiver is shown in figure 15.

The signal from the probe is only of the order of microvolts. It is therefore essential that the preamplifier introduces very little additional noise. The function of the preamplifier and the main amplifier is to boost the received signal without any adverse effects on the SNR. Further, the very sensitive preamplifier must be protected from the high power transmitter pulse. To this end, in cross-coil systems for example, a group of crossed diodes are introduced in series in the transmitter line to improve the ring-down during the radiofrequency pulse and to reduce transmitter noise during signal reception. Similarly, crossed diodes are placed in parallel with the input to the preamplifier to protect this device from overload during the radio-frequency pulse arising from imperfect orthogonality of the receiver and transmitter coils.

The overall gain of the receiver amplifiers is $\sim 10^5$; thus the output signal is typically a few volts. This signal is then fed into one or more phase sensitive detectors whose output can be shown to be of the form $\cos[(\omega_0 - \omega_s)t + \phi]$, where ω_s is the signal frequency and ω_0 is the frequency of a reference. The reference is normally chosen to be the centre frequency with which the sample was irradiated. The NMR signal has therefore been converted to an audio signal with a bandwidth of a few kHz.

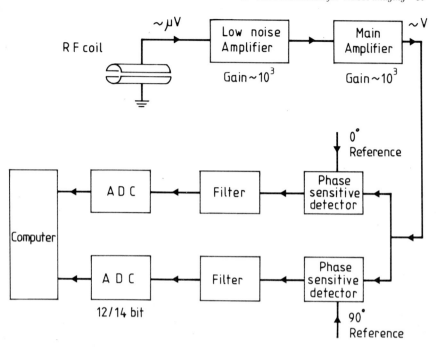

Figure 15. A schematic diagram of the NMR receiver.

When a single phase sensitive detector is used information is lost as to whether $(\omega_0 - \omega_s)$ is positive or negative. Following Fourier transformation all signals will therefore appear to one side of the reference frequency regardless of the sign of $(\omega_0 - \omega_s)$. If such a system is used care must be taken to ensure that ω_0 is set at a frequency either higher or lower than all the information frequencies. Similarly, noise is reflected about the reference frequency and two sets of noise contribute to the spectrum instead of one. Since noise is random, this causes the noise amplitude to increase by a factor of $\sqrt{2}$ and SNR to decrease by a factor of $\sqrt{2}$.

The use of two phase sensitive detectors detecting in quadrature (i.e., the phase of the reference is shifted by $90°$ in one of the detectors) permits the separation of positive and negative frequencies on Fourier transformation. As a result there is an improvement in the SNR by a factor of $\sqrt{2}$. The phase sensitive detected signals are then fed to low pass filters before digitization.

2.7. The computer system

As we have seen, it is convenient to separate the control function from the data processing. We have used a microcomputer for gradient and radiofrequency pulse control. However, care must be taken with synchronization of the various elements of the pulse sequence, i.e., gradients and pulses. In general, it is not possible to achieve the required accuracy purely by software means. In our system, the microcomputer is used to load external memory and timers with appropriate values and to enable and disable circuit elements as required. The use of high frequency counters permits accurate timing and the output of functions from external hardware is readily synchronized.

Data is collected via one or more analogue to digital convertors (ADCs). These must normally be followed by a buffer memory, as the computer system is often too slow to accept the data direct. We have used a 10 bit Data Laboratory's Transient Recorder for this purpose. However, a 12 bit ADC is preferable due to the large dynamic range of the data, and 12 bit ADCs of sufficient speed are now commercially available. For a signal bandwidth of say 10 kHz, a sampling interval of 50 µs or less is required to satisfy the Nyquist theorem. This assumes that we have a perfect rectangular low pass filter of bandwidth 10 kHz. In practice it is not possible to achieve such a sharp cut-off. Under the conditions described above, high frequency noise would be undersampled and would therefore fold back onto the signal frequencies: this is called aliasing. To overcome this problem, the sampling rate is increased sufficiently to resolve correctly all frequencies that are passed by the filter. The high frequency noise is then discarded after Fourier transformation.

The main computer system must perform the functions of (i) collection of data from the buffer memory, (ii) Fourier transformation, (iii) phase correction from imperfect setting up of the pulse sequence and from the phase response of the low pass filter, (iv) the display of time and frequency data, (v) image reconstruction, (vi) image display, and (vii) interactive image processing. Finally there must be some means of mass data storage available.

For rapid data processing an array processor or hardware Fast Fourier Transform unit are a considerable advantage. In the absence of either of these facilities a computer system with a 24 or 32 bit word length will permit integer arithmetic written in Assembly language to give optimum data processing time. In addition a large main computer memory is required so that the raw data and processed image arrays may be stored simultaneously. Considerable time may be lost in writing and retrieving data to and from storage media such as discs and magnetic tapes. The image display normally has its own dedicated external memory and will be capable of displaying up to 256 pixel square 8 bit images.

References

1. Brigham E O 1974 *The Fast Fourier Transform* (London: Prentice-Hall)
2. Hoult D I 1977 Zeugmatography: A criticism of the concept of a selective pulse in the presence of a field gradient *Journal of Magnetic Resonance* **26** 165–7
3. Sutherland R J and Hutchison J M S 1978 Three dimensional NMR imaging using selective excitation *Journal of Physics E: Scientific Instruments* **11** 79–83

4. Mansfield P, Maudsley A A, Morris P G and Pykett I L 1979 Selective pulses in NMR imaging: A repy to criticism *Journal of Magnetic Resonance* **33** 261–74
5. Mansfield P and Morris P G 1982 *NMR Imaging in Biomedicine* (London: Academic Press)
6. Gadian D G 1982 *Nuclear Magnetic Resonance and its Applications to Living Systems* (Oxford University Press)
7. Zupančič and Pirš J 1976 Coils producing a magnetic field gradient for diffusion measurements with NMR *Journal of Physics E: Scientific Instruments* **9** 79–80
8. Hoult D I 1981 Radio frequency coil technology in NMR scanning *Proceedings of International Symposium on NMR Imaging, Winston-Salem, USA* (Bowman Gray School of Medicine Press)
9. Hoult D I and Richards R E 1976 The signal-to-noise ratio of the Nuclear Magnetic Resonance Experiment *Journal of Magnetic Resonance* **24** 71–85
10. Hoult D I and Lauterbur P C 1979 The sensitivity of the zeugmatographic experiment involving human samples *Journal of Magnetic Resonance* **34** 425–33
11. Hoult D I 1978 The NMR receiver: A description and analysis of design *Progress in Nuclear Magnetic Resonance Spectroscopy* **12** 41–77

CHAPTER **3 An introduction to magnet design and operation**
W E Timms

Oxford Research Systems Limited, Nuffield Way,
Abingdon, Oxon OX14 1RY, England

3.1. General introduction

At the heart of any NMR system is a volume of space containing a uniform magnetic field. The first part of this paper sets out a framework of NMR terms in which to describe the magnet and its detailed operation by the user. The remainder of the paper is divided into two parts. The first of these (sections 3.2 and 3.3) is mostly descriptive and deals very briefly with the practical aspects of day to day running of a magnet. The second (section 3.4) covers design and analysis and links the concepts of the first part with the mathematical and physical descriptions of the magnet.

When magnets are described it is assumed that they will have been designed with easy and comfortable access for a human subject. For large resistive magnets and superconducting magnets, this demands a horizontal multisolenoidal coil design and some sort of patient carrier or bed running parallel to the axis (and hence the field) of the solenoid. The smaller resistive magnets and the permanent magnets can have patient access transverse to the field direction. This can give some practical advantages in the design of the radio frequency coils used for signal acquisition.

To reduce the length of the introduction to NMR, reference will be made to other sources and only the basic results will be introduced. Where it is relevant a small amount of explanation will be offered which will, hopefully, link the NMR concepts to those understood by the average physicist (or magnet designer) who requires a system which is easy to operate.

3.2. Concepts and practical points

3.2.1. Basic NMR and field homogeneity

As explained in other literature [1-5], the NMR experiment can only work on nuclei which have non-zero spin. Such nuclei also have a magnetic moment the energy of which will vary with its orientation to an external magnetic field. The ratio of the moment to the spin is characteristic of the nuclear species.

Quantum mechanics requires any changes in spin to have only integer values, thus generating a series of energy levels for the magnetic moment. A "spin one" change in energy levels of a magnetic moment is accompanied by the radiation or absorption of a quantum of electromagnetic radiation (typically in the radiofrequency (RF) region). In NMR the relationships are expressed as

$$\omega_0 = \gamma B_0 \tag{1}$$

where ω_0 ($= 2\pi f_0$) is the angular frequency of the RF and B_0 is the applied magnetic induction. The constant γ is the gyromagnetic ratio, typical of the nuclear type, and represents the ratio of the moment to the spin. Equation (1) is not obviously a quantum mechanical expression but as can be seen in the references, it does represent the quantum processes involved in the "spin-one" transitions. For a particular nuclear type the value of the applied field of B_0 can vary slightly depending upon the chemical environment of the atom containing the nucleus. This effect is the "chemical shift" and can be used to identify the chemical environment, its value varies from a few parts in 10^{10} up to several hundred parts in 10^6 of the mean value.

If the interaction between a nucleus in a magnetic field, B_0, and an RF wave is studied it is found that there is resonant absorption over a range of frequencies close to ω_0. This is in the form of an absorption line of Lorentzian shape

$$f(\omega) = \frac{\Delta_0^2}{(\omega - \omega_0)^2 + \Delta_0^2} \tag{2}$$

where $2\Delta_0$ is the width of the line at half height. The source of this linewidth is the interaction between the nuclei, which causes stimulated emission and absorption. This process is typified by a life time T_2 of the nuclear spin states which is equal to the inverse of Δ_0.

When the B_0 field is not uniform then ω_0 varies across the system of nuclei giving a superposition of lines described by equation (2), each weighted by the number of nuclei in the particular field value. The effect of this can be approximated by an increased value Δ_0 which depends upon the field distribution across the whole sample of nuclei. The corresponding combined time constant is T_2^*. It is interesting to point out that this problem of line broadening gives hints of the technique of imaging which utilizes controlled variation of field across the sample.

In the early days of NMR the method of measurement was the obvious one of sweeping the value of one parameter (frequency or field) and measuring the absorption of RF energy, and was called the continuous wave method (CW). With the advent of high speed computer controlled data acquisition systems the CW method has given way to the much more powerful method that measures the response function of the nuclei to an impulse excitation. The measured response is a time varying signal which is radiated by the nuclei (called a free induction decay or FID) after the impulse. The envelope of the FID is an exponential decay with time constant T_2^* whilst the detailed structure of the FID contains only information about the frequency of the spectral lines corresponding to the different nuclear species.

Since T_2^* is less than T_2 and because this difference comes from field inhomogeneity across the sample of nuclei, there is available a simple method of increasing the field homogeneity. Small changes can be made to the field distribution and improvements observed by increasing the time constant T_2^*, i.e., the FID persists for longer and becomes "fatter". This process is known as shimming and is usually done by changing the currents in specially designed coils known (not surprisingly) as shim coils. The field can also be shimmed by the more difficult process of placing small pieces of iron near the magnet. To obtain the spectrum the FID is Fourier transformed and displayed by the computer. Figure 1 shows the spectra obtained from a well shimmed and

(a)

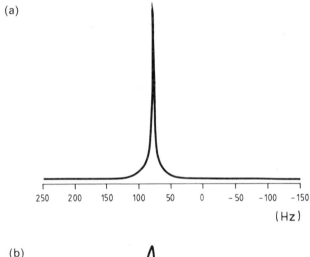

(b)

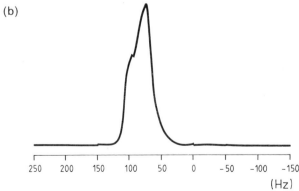

Figure 1. (a) Proton spectrum of a 40 mm diameter sphere of water, shimmed to 3.5 Hz line width at half height. (b) The same sphere in the presence of an X-gradient. (The vertical scale is expanded by a factor of four.)

a badly shimmed sphere of water. Notice that the latter is of smaller amplitude than the former and shows structure indicative of the field distribution across the sphere. The integrated area under both lines is the same and is a measure of the number of nuclei present in the sphere. The same information is also present in the FID and is represented by the amplitude at "zero" time after the impulse. Consequently this amplitude does not change during shimming.

One more point needs introducing into this practical résumé, namely the spin–lattice relaxation time T_1. This is equal to or longer than T_2 and measures the time constant of the processes which remove the impulse energy from the nuclei and transfer it to the surrounding "lattice" of atoms. It should be emphasized that T_1 is not the same as T_2, which only measures the time constant for redistribution of energy amongst the nuclei. Thus after an impulse when the FID has disappeared the sample may still not be in the state it was before the impulse. In practice it is necessary to wait a time at least $5T_1$ before repeating the experiment. Too rapid a repetition varies the total amplitude of the FIDs, which can make shimming impossible. The whole effect is known as "saturation" of the nuclear spin system.

3.2.2. Application in spectroscopy

As the name implies, NMR spectroscopy generates a spectrum of frequencies of a particular nuclear species with the intention of analysing the chemical shifts and signal amplitudes (or areas) to give relative concentrations of identified chemicals.

The accuracy with which this can be done depends upon the accuracies with which the frequency and area of the spectral lines can be measured. The best positional accuracy is obtained when the lines are narrowest and separated by the largest amount. Narrowness is limited by T_2 in a perfect magnet and T_2 is usually independent of B_0. The separation is, however, linearly proportional to B_0 so that the best resolution is usually obtained at the highest fields.

There is a further, and very important, reason for working at high fields, namely that the signal strength of the FID increases with some power of B_0 in the range 1.0 to 1.75. This increases the received signal-to-noise ratio since the noise power per unit bandwidth is substantially constant. The practical limits on B_0 tend to come from the radiofrequency (RF) skin depth when applied to typical human body dimensions. This limit at present is in the region of $2T$ and is close to the financial/technical limits that manufacturers and customers are prepared to tolerate.

Table 1 gives the typical requirements of a spectroscopy magnet compared with an imaging magnet. The smaller but more uniform volume of field for spectroscopy is necessary because localized chemical analysis is the requirement for clinical purposes. It is evident however that a well designed high field imaging magnet could also meet the criteria for spectroscopy.

Table 1. The design criteria for magnets used in the three main applications of NMR to medicine. A high resolution analytical spectrometer gives *in vitro* spectra of tissue samples or extracts of the tissue.

Application	Imaging	*In vivo* spectroscopy	High resolution analytical spectrometer
Field	0.05 T upwards	1–2 T	1–15 T Axis usually vertical
Homogeneous volume	Whole-body section, 200–500 mm diameter sphere or cylinder	Internal organ or muscle size, ∼50 mm diameter sphere	5–25 mm diameter cylinder, by 10–25 mm long
Field homogeneity	10 ppm	0.1 ppm	5 parts in 10^9 to 1 part in 10^{10}
Special notes	1. Static patient 2. Pulsed field gradients	1. Move patient to bring target to centre 2. "Shim" the field	1. Sample taken and placed in a standard "sample tube". 2. "Shim" the field. 3. Spin the sample tube about its axis.

For more detailed information on applications the reader should see references 1 to 6 and the contribution of Radda *et al.* in reference 11. (Reference 6 contains a longer list of references to *in vivo* techniques). A more descriptive paper by Shulman[7] also gives an interesting introduction to uses of *in vivo* spectroscopy.

3.2.3. Application in imaging

The computer algorithm used to process the data acquired during an investigation (a period of time between 0.5 and 20 min) makes the assumptions that the field B_0 is uniform and constant and that the gradients are linear and reproducible. Any variation from these conditions will cause the data to be assigned to the wrong parts of the image. The design of an imaging magnet system will require knowledge of the real variations in field etc. so that the other available parameters can be chosen for best image quality. This means that a poor B_0 homogeneity or stability requires larger values of gradient and a wider RF bandwidth for the signal receiving system. The result of this is satisfactory image definition but a reduced signal-to-noise ratio. In practice the maximum realizable gradients in a one metre bore magnet are about 0.8 G cm^{-1} with the limit imposed by coil and power supply design.

Table 1 gives typical operating requirements for an imaging system for whole body studies. For further reading the references 8 to 11 are suggested. A descriptive introduction to imaging can be found in reference 12.

3.3. Magnet types

3.3.1. Introduction

At present three types of magnet are being considered for use in the clinical NMR systems of the future. Over the next five years the merits and drawbacks of these competing types are likely to be fully determined and one or more "standard" configuration may become pre-eminent. Since the demand for NMR systems is likely to fall into the two broad classes of "routine" and "research" there may be a natural division of magnet types with the research requirement being satisfied by a versatile, high-field superconducting magnet. The more routine instruments will probably use either a lower field super-conducting magnet, a resistive multicoil electromagnet or a permanent magnet.

The description of these various magnet types, their operation and peculiarities has been discussed recently by Gordon and Timms[13] and so this section will only be a very brief introduction to the choice of magnet. In the above article it is emphasized that the whole magnet site should be carefully planned in order to gain optimum magnet performance and safety. The safety aspect is relatively simple to plan but care must be taken over the correct day to day operation to control unauthorized access to the magnet. This rather pedantic attitude to magnet safety is a result of the author's experience with various peoples' appreciation of the risks. The situation is best summed up by saying that the effects of a strong magnetic field are totally beyond most people's intuition and can not be classed as "common sense".

3.3.2. Permanent magnets

The operating conditions for these magnets are the least understood by the NMR community, but those operators familiar with the small analytical spectrometers using permanent magnets, will know that the simplicity of operation can be an illusion. When scaled up to whole-body size the problems are the same, in addition to those posed by the pulsed gradient coil require-ment. The author has no knowledge of the response of the magnet to these pulses and can give no guidance to a user.

The strength of their magnetic field limits permanent magnets to the imaging method where any instabilities are relatively unimportant. There is an advantage on a site with restricted size because the peripheral field of the system is much less than that of a comparable electromagnet.

3.3.3. Resistive electromagnets

These magnets really *look* like high power magnets with big water cooled coils supplying the field. Their operation is simple and straightforward once the temperature has stabilized. Typical field values are up to 0.15 or 0.2 T for an electrical imput power of 60 kW to 100 kW, depending upon the actual design.

An extension of this type is the iron augmented electromagnet which has an external iron case to provide the return path for the magnetic flux which passes through the bore of the magnet. In this design approximately 20% of the field comes from the iron, thus giving a significant reduction in the power consumption. Alternatively, for the same power, the maximum field can reach 0.25 T. A further advantage over the simple electromagnet is a reduction in the peripheral field.

3.3.4. Superconducting magnets

Of all the magnet types the superconducting magnet, built into its cryostat, looks the most innocuous. There are no heavy current leads present nor cooling water when the magnet is energized and in persistent mode. Apart from the size of the instrument there is no indication of the very powerful field that may be present. This field spreads for large distances and may require the shielding of nearby equipment.

The current generation of the cryostat uses liquid helium and liquid nitrogen to keep the magnet superconducting. These should have daily level checks and will typically require refilling with helium every month and with nitrogen every week. Future generations of cryostat will undoubtedly incorporate mechanical cooling engines to extend the refill period and perhaps to eliminate the liquid nitrogen requirement. The expected helium refill period will probably lie between six months and one year, with an annual service for the engine. This performance could lead to a full service contract where the user does not have to worry about the cryogen refill.

A speculative point should be made at this time concerning helium as a scarce natural resource. The commercial sources of helium gas are oil wells and natural gas wells in certain parts of the world, and these have political and production restraints. It is generally believed in the cryogenic community that these sources of helium will be severely depleted sometime after the year 2000 and that there will be very practical reasons for the conservation of helium stocks. This aim will be helped by the introduction of cooling engines and may eventually lead to the "closed cycle" cryostat with recycled helium.

3.4. Magnetic field analysis and stability

3.4.1. Introduction

In section 3.2 it was shown how the different NMR techniques require different homogeneity of magnetic field; section 3.4 deals with the mathematical analysis of the field in the region occupied by the experiment and outside the magnet. The sources of stress in the magnet structure are described and discussed in the case of solenoidal magnets. The more complex cases of permanent magnets or iron augmented magnets are introduced at a level sufficient to show the real design problems. Finally the various sources of field instability are identified and quantified.

3.4.2. Near magnet centre

This is the region of primary importance to the magnet user and is best kept clear of all field sources that may affect the homogeneity or value of the magnetic field. In practice this means that there are no loops carrying circulating currents and no magnetizable materials within this region.

Maxwell's equations[14, 15] thus give

$$\text{curl } \boldsymbol{B} = 0 \tag{3}$$

which has a particular solution for the z-axis field component given by

$$
\begin{aligned}
B_z = B_0 + \sum_{n=0}^{\infty} r^n \{ & A_n P_n(\mu) \\
& + \sum_{m=1}^{n} C_{nm} P_n^m(\mu) \exp[\mathrm{j}(m\phi + \xi_{nm})] \}
\end{aligned}
\tag{4}
$$

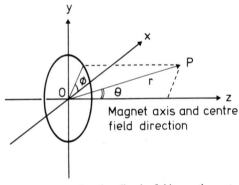

Figure 2.   The coordinate system used to describe the field near the centre of a magnet. The measuring point (P) is denoted by the spherical coordinates (r, θ, ϕ), measured from magnet centre (O), which are equivalent to the Cartesian coordinates (x, y, z).

where A_n and C_{nm} are undetermined constants and ξ_{nm} is a phase constant. The coordinate system is shown in figure 2. $P_n(\mu)$ and $P_n^m(\mu)$ are respectively Legendre and Associated Legendre functions, and $\mu = \cos \theta$. The solution set with $n \geqslant 0$ has been chosen since it represents the real situation with a constant centre field, B_0, and various "impurities" which increase with the distance from the centre. In fact the solution is only valid within a radius R, which is the distance from the centre of the closest source coil or magnetizable object. As r approaches R so the number of terms required in equation (4) increases in order to express the field to a given accuracy.

Starting with a current element and the Biot–Savart law[14, 15] equation (4) can be derived and the constants A_n and C_{nm} evaluated. For a circular arc of radius a_0, centred on the z-axis it is found that these constants can be separated in terms of the arc coordinates to give

$$A_n = F_n/a_0^{n+1} \tag{5a}$$

and

$$C_{nm} = G_{nm}/a_0^{n+1} \tag{5b}$$

where F and G are functions only of the angular positions of the source arcs.

If the terms in equation (4) are turned into Cartesian coordinates it is found that for $n = 1$

$$A_1 r P_1(\mu) = A_1 z \tag{6a}$$

and

$$C_{11} r P_1(\mu) \cos(\phi + \xi_{11}) = S_{11} x + T_{11} y \tag{6b}$$

where S_{11} and T_{11} are constants. These terms are simply the linear gradients that can occur and which are deliberately generated for imaging. The higher order terms in n and m give rise to "impurities" which vary with higher powers of x, y and z.

The formulation of equation (4) is very convenient for design purposes because each term splits neatly into the product of a measuring point term and a source term. This allows the various coils of a magnet to be treated individually and their contributions to equation (4) to be summed. The design objective is to reduce all the constants A_n and C_{nm} to zero for $n \leqslant N$ and to make the remaining terms smaller than the chosen design criterion for the required volume near the magnet centre.

The lowest order term, B_0, is usually treated in a different fashion to the other terms because of the required accuracy. The simplest example is for a thick solenoid of length $2l$, inner radius a and outer radius b, carrying a current density J (metric units). Then the field at the centre of the solenoid is given by

$$B_0 = J a \mu_0 F(\alpha, \beta) \tag{7}$$

where

$$F(\alpha, \beta) = \beta \ln\left(\frac{\alpha + (\alpha^2 + \beta^2)^{\frac{1}{2}}}{1 + (1 + \beta^2)^{\frac{1}{2}}}\right) \tag{8}$$

and $\alpha = b/a$, $\beta = l/a$. μ_0 is the permeability of free space $(-4\pi \times 10^{-7} \text{ H m}^{-1})$. To describe the field at any other point on the axis a simple modification of equations (7) and (8) can be derived.

When a magnet is made from real materials (as against the perfect materials assumed during the design), and when it is placed in the magnetic environment of a real building it is not surprising to find that the field is no longer perfectly homogeneous but contains many of the terms of equation (4). If the magnet design is good and the effects of the building checked before placing the magnet then the principal inhomogeneities will correspond to small values of n with the terms containing high n values becoming quickly insignificant.

This is the point of contact between magnet design and shim coil design. Once the former is fixed the probable values of field inhomogeneity can be estimated, and thus the strengths of the shim coils are determined. The design of shim coils has been discussed[16-18] and several geometries of coil have been produced. Simplest amongst them are those that can be wound or assembled on a cylindrical coil former.

Symmetry arguments show that the most efficient designs for axial shims (those associated with A_n in equation (4)) are constructed from circular coils wound onto the cylinder. The numbers of turns in each coil and their positions along the axis allow a set of coils to produce only one of the terms in $P_n(\mu)$ with any significant strength over the working volume of the magnet. In general, the larger the diameter of this volume with respect to the winding diameter of the coils, the more difficult it is to produce a "pure" shim.

Shims which produce transverse variations of the B_0 field always occur in pairs, each of the same design, but offset from each other by an angle determined by m in equation (4). (Two shim coils are required because there are two transverse dimensions.) These are again designed to produce only one significant term in P_n^m. The simplest designs are constructed from arcs of circles on the cylinder, joined together by wires parallel to the axis. Only the arcs need to be considered in the calculations since the axial wires produce no z-component of the field. The transverse field of such coils can generally be ignored at the level of homogeneity required for *in vivo* spectroscopy, but not necessarily at the level required for high resolution *in vitro* chemical analysis spectrometers.

The arc lengths and positions can be derived from the Biot–Savart law and by considering the mathematical symmetry of the required shim functions. For a more detailed description of these designs see the references 16 to 18 and the references therein.

3.4.3. Fields and forces on the magnet

The magnetic fields and forces acting on the windings of the magnet are of little interest to the average user. Nevertheless, to ensure safety and correct operation of the magnet these parameters must be calculated and demonstrated to be in the correct operational areas. Superconducting magnets have constraints additional to those of ordinary resistive magnets. Initially the common criteria will be discussed.

The forces on an energized simple solenoid can be visualized as having two physical effects. One tries to compress the solenoid along its axis whilst the other tries to burst the solenoid by pushing the windings outwards. Obviously these effects will vary from place to place within the solenoid. The source of the forces is the usual "electric-motor" force. Thus if J is the local current density (A m^{-2}) and B is the local magnetic induction (tesla) then the local force is

$$F = J \times B \tag{9}$$

In a solenoid the current is azimuthal and B has only axial (B_z) and radial (B_ρ) components. Hence the force (per metre of wire) has only axial and radial components given by

$$F_z = JB_\rho \tag{10a}$$

and

$$F_\rho = JB_z \tag{10b}$$

Considering the symmetry of a simple solenoid and the dipole field that it generates, B_z is nearly always in the same direction in the windings, thus F_ρ is always outwards. On the mid-plane B_ρ is zero and changes sign, thus giving opposite signed forces on each side of the middle.

The radial force acting outwards against the curved windings (of radius r) produces a tension (S) in the wire known as the hoop stress

$$S = rJB_z \text{ (N m}^{-2}) \tag{11}$$

There will be some limiting value of S beyond which the solenoid will not work or will be unsafe. Consequently, as magnets are made bigger, the value of the product JB_z must be reduced to prevent failure.

The axial compressive force is not quite such a problem since it is easier to contain, but it can not be ignored. Typically on a large, high-field magnet superconducting solenoid there will be a total compressive force of well over 100 tonnes (10^5 kg).

In general, large NMR magnets are formed from more than one solenoid section, linked electrically and mechanically together. Here the forces and fields are not simple and it is possible, for instance, that the hoop stress may change sign within the depth of a winding. To maintain the designed high homogeneity of the central field it is necessary to ensure that the linking structures are not significantly strained by the inter-coil forces. Whenever possible the best stress analysis of the magnet system should be carried out.

To calculate the fields on the magnet windings it is again necessary to resort to the Biot–Savart law and integrate the effects of the whole magnet. Fortunately, over the years, this problem has been well investigated by many authors and most of the geometries encountered in the design of NMR magnets have been considered and analytical or calculable solutions derived[17, 19, 20]. For solenoids and assemblies of solenoids the calculations require nothing more difficult than complete elliptic integrals. The most useful collection of formulae and equations has been made by Garrett[20] and makes a designer's life considerably simpler!

Returning now to superconducting magnets, these have all the problems discussed above, usually in a more severe form than a resistive magnet. The reason for this is simply that the superconducting magnets have to produce significantly higher fields in an equally large volume of space. The additional problems arise because of the intrinsic properties of superconducting wires, which limit the current density J as a function of B. The relationship is not simple and requires the designer to make a decision on the operating conditions for the magnet, based on experience and the will to remain employed.

The type of superconductor used also has properties which are a bit remote from common experience. Although a constant current can flow in it without resistive loss, a changing current can dissipate energy as heat. This is also taken into account during the design since this process can limit the rate at which a superconducting magnet can be brought to full field.

The last point of consideration is the way in which every element of superconducting wire must be fully immobilized during construction. If a small element of wire moves by only fractions of a millimetre or breaks away from its fixed position then a quantity of heat is generated. Although this is very small, the specific heat of the wire at 4.2 K is, by comparison, negligible and a significant temperature increase can occur. This causes a reduction in the safe current density leading to more heating. The heating spreads rapidly through the windings and quickly dissipates the magnetic field energy as heat—this evaporates the liquid helium giving the well known visual and sound effects of a "quench".

3.4.4. Distant fields

The distant field and its gradient are of real interest because of their nuisance values and for safety of the general public. Their calculation is straight-forward using the elliptic integral method mentioned in the last section. The prime safety factors which must be considered are listed briefly below. Some are direct whilst others are indirect and more subtle in the dangers that they might cause.

(i) Cardiac pacemakers

These have a test mode which is activated by a magnetic reed-relay switch. Experiments performed at Oxford Research Systems on a UK manufactured device and on a USA manufactured device showed that the UK device was activated above about 20 G (1600 A m^{-1}) whilst the USA device switched at a range of values above 5.5 G (440 A m^{-1}). These are the only data available to the author and are not the result of large statistical tests. It seems to be generally agreed that a figure of 5 G (400 A m^{-1}) should not be exceeded in any area which can be entered by the general public without positive vetting by a qualified person.

(ii) Mechanical force

This results from the magnetic attraction of iron or steel towards the magnet. This force is mostly caused by the magnetization of the steel and the gradient of the magnetic field. The former is somewhat dependent on the material and the latter can be easily calculated. As a rough rule of thumb the force on an object is the same as its weight somewhere near the 100 G contour and varies approximately as the inverse fourth power of distance from the magnet.

(iii) Interference with other analytical systems

If the peripheral field of the magnet affects nearby apparatus there is a possibility of mis-analysis by the apparatus. If the result leads to clinical or drug treatment then the interference should be classed as dangerous. A more detailed treatment of the safety aspects and site planning has been made by Gordon and Timms[13] and is also referred to in the literature of various system manufacturers.

3.4.5. Magnetizable materials

Since magnetizable materials such as iron and steel are non-linear in their response to a magnetic field, it is not possible to write down an analytical solution to a general system of field sources and magnetic material. Instead, numerical solutions must be sought with the aid of computer programs. This in itself is a large subject fraught with difficulties.

If we have a system of field sources which alone produce a field variation $H_s(r)$ as a function of position r and then introduce the magnetizable material, then the local magnetization $M(r^1)$ within the material must be solved in some way to generate the total local field $H(r)$. The iteration loop is closed by the "known" relationship between the local susceptibility χ and H

$$M(r^1) = \chi(|H|)H(r^1) \tag{12}$$

and

$$H(r) = H_0(r) - \nabla \int M(r^1) \cdot \nabla(1/R)\,dV \tag{13}$$

Here $R = r^1 - r$ and the integral is over the volume of magnetizable material. These problems and their solution are discussed in more detail in references 21 to 23.

3.4.6. Stability (electrical and thermal)

For electromagnets the electrical stability is determined by the required field stability. For an imaging magnet this will be a small fraction of the field variation that covers one picture element. Thus working at 0.3 G cm^{-1} and a picture element size of (say) 2 mm then the field per element is 0.06 G. If the mixing of element data is to be less than 5% then the field stability (from all sources) is to be better than 3 mG. For a 1.5 kG magnet this represents 2 parts per million (ppm) of field and current stability during an experiment. This is at the very limit of the best power supply stability and is not normally to be expected. For a superconducting magnet in persistent mode this should not be a problem since field decay rates are normally less than 0.1 ppm h^{-1}.

The data on permanent magnets and their materials is not readily available, but the temperature coefficients of the materials suggest a worse stability than the resistive electromagnet. This type of instability would however give a slow change because of the thermal inertia of the mass of metal.

Dimensional stability is not a problem for superconducting magnets since they are extremely isothermal under normal operating conditions and the thermal expansion coefficient is very close to zero! This is not true, however, for a permanent magnet or for a resistive solenoid, and an analysis of the latter indicates the required temperature control.

Consider a magnet designed such that only B_0 is significant in equation (4). The value of B_0 is proportional to the number of ampere turns in the windings and inversely proportional to the radius on which the coils are wound

$$B_0 \propto NI/a_0 \tag{14}$$

thus

$$\frac{\delta B_0}{B_0} = \frac{-\delta a_0}{a_0} \tag{15}$$

where δB_0 and δa_0 are corresponding small changes in B_0 and a_0. If the source of δa_0 is thermal expansion due to a change δT in temperature then

$$\delta a_0/a_0 = \delta T \cdot \zeta \tag{16}$$

where ζ is the coefficient of linear expansion (1.7×10^{-5} °C^{-1} for copper and 2.3×10^{-5} °C^{-1} for aluminium). Hence for an aluminium structure requiring 1 ppm stability, $\delta T < 0.04$ °C. In a magnet subject to water cooling, forced and convected air cooling and a total heat load of 60 kW in 2 tonnes of metal, such stability is surprising at first sight but not unreasonable after a settling time has been allowed. (Without cooling the rate of temperature increase would be about 0.03 °C s^{-1}.)

If different support materials are used to space the magnet coils from each other, or the supports are at different temperatures to the windings, then the balance of coefficients in equations (4) and (5) will be upset, thus introducing unwanted field gradients. These must be shimmed out after the settling time.

3.5. Other considerations and conclusions

So far the design and operation of magnets has been discussed with respect to NMR applications. To complete the picture of the total system the various safety regulations should be introduced. These cover the user's site, the system design and user modifications to the equipment. Gordon and Timms[13] give a personalized view of these regulations but the definitive sources are references such as 24 to 31 which have been generated by national and international standards organizations.

The technique of NMR when applied to living human subjects is inherently safe, and all investigations for harmful effects have given negative results to date. References 24 and 25 put certain limits on the NMR parameters, but go on to explain that these are based upon "noticeable" effects and not on danger levels. It is likely that most danger will come from magnetic materials being allowed too close to the magnet by inadequately trained personnel. The hospital environment is already used to coping with dangerous diagnostic and therapeutic x-ray systems, and so with similar safeguards the NMR systems will become a routine investigative tool.

3.6. Acknowledgements

I am indebted to my co-workers at Oxford Research Systems for comments and advice and in particular to Dr R E Gordon for checking the clarity of presentation.

Thanks are also due to Dr G K Radda, Dr P J Bore and Mr P Styles of the Medical Research Council Clinical Magnetic Research Laboratory at the John Radcliffe Hospital, for comments and discussions concerning the application of NMR techniques to human subjects.

References

1. Farrar T C and Becker E D 1971 *Pulse and Fourier Transform NMR* (New York: Academic Press)
2. Abragam A 1971 *The Principles of Nuclear Magnetism*, revised edn (Oxford University Press)
3. Fukushima E and Roeder S B W 1981 *Experimental Pulse NMR: A Nuts and Bolts Approach* (New York: Addison-Wesley)
4. McFarlane W and White R F M 1972 *Techniques of High Resolution Nuclear Magnetic Resonance* (London: Butterworths)
5. Müllen K and Pregosin P S 1976 *Fourier Transform NMR Techniques: A practical approach* (New York: Academic Press)
6. Gadian D G 1982 *Nuclear Magnetic Resonance and its Applications to Living Systems* (Oxford University Press)
7. Shulman R G 1983 NMR spectroscopy of living cells, *Scientific American* **248** (1) 76–83
8. Lauterbur P C 1973 Image formation by induced local interactions *Nature* **242** 190–191
9. Pykett I L, Buonanno F S, Brady T J and Kistler J P 1983 Techniques and approaches to proton NMR imaging of the head *Computerized Radiology* **7** 1–18
10. Kaufman L, Crooks L E and Margulis A R (eds) 1981 *Nuclear Magnetic Resonance Imaging* (Tokyo: Igaku-Shoin)

11. Karstaedt N, Witcofski R L and Partain C L (eds) 1982 *Proceedings of an International Symposium on NMR Imaging* (Winston-Salem, N C: Bowman Gray School of Medicine Press)
12. Pykett I L 1982 NMR Imaging in Medicine *Scientific American* **246** (5) 54–64
13. Gordon R E and Timms W E 1984 *Computerized Radiology* **8** (5)
14. Bleaney B I and Bleaney B 1965 *Electricity and Magnetism* 2nd edn (Oxford University Press)
15. Jackson J D 1975 *Classical Electrodynamics* (Chichester: John Wiley)
16. Golay M J E 1958 *Review of Scientific Instruments* **29** 313
17. Garrett M W 1967 *Journal of Applied Physics* **38** 2563
18. Roméo F and Hoult D I 1984 *Magnetic Resonance in Medicine* **1** 44–65
19. Wilson M N 1983 *Superconducting Magnets* (Oxford University Press)
20. Garrett M W 1965 *Oak Ridge National Laboratory Publication* ORNL-3575
21. Armstrong A G, Collie C J, Simkin J and Trowbridge C W 1978 The solution of 3D magnetostatic problems using scalar potentials. In *Proceedings of COMPUMAG 2 Conference, Grenoble* (Laboratoire de Electrotechnique, ENSEGP, BT 46, 38402 St Martin d'Heres, France)
22. *Rutherford Laboratory publication* RL-81-076, 1981 (Part of proceedings of COMPUMAG conference at Chicago)
23. Simkin J and Trowbridge C W 1980 Three-dimensional non-linear electromagnetic computations using scalar potentials, *IEE Proceedings* **127** (B6) 368–374
24. National Radiological Protection Board (UK) 1981 Exposure to nuclear magnetic resonance clinical imaging *Radiography* **47** 258–260
25. Food and Drug Administration (USA) 1982 *Guidelines for evaluating electromagnetic exposure risk for trials of clinical NMR systems* (Washington, DC: Public Health Service)
26. International Electrotechnical Commission 1977 *Safety of medical electrical equipment, Part 1: General Requirements* (IEC 601-1)
27. British Standards Institution 1979 *Safety of medical electrical equipment: General Requirements* BS 5724, Part 1 (This is a British standard, almost identical to IEC 601, part 1)
28. UL544 1981 *Standard for Medical and Dental Requirement* (Published by Underwriters Laboratories Inc, Northbrook, Illinois 60062, USA)
29. DHSS 1981 *Technical Requirements for the Supply and Installation of NMR Apparatus (1981)* TRS 81 (Published by the Department of Health and Social Security, Scientific and Technical Branch (STB6A) in the United Kingdom)
30. British Standards Institution *Unfired, fusion welded pressure vessels* BS 5500 (This is a British Standard for pressure vessels and is more suited to cryostat construction than the pressure vessel specifications of IEC 601 part 1)
31. *ASME Boiler and Pressure Vessel Code*, Section VIII *Unfired Pressure Vessels* (American Society of Mechanical Engineers)

R A Lerski

Department of Medical Physics, Hammersmith Hospital,
Du Cane Road, London W12 0HS, England

4.1. Introduction

The basic nuclear magnetic resonance (NMR) experiment is performed by placing the sample of interest in a very uniform magnetic field, conventionally in the Z direction, and disturbing the equilibrium nuclear magnetization through applied radiofrequency RF pulses at the Larmor frequency (figure 1). A free induction decay (FID) signal may be received as the magnetization relaxes back to equilibrium and this signal will again be at the Larmor frequency

$$\omega_0 = \gamma \boldsymbol{B}_0 \tag{1}$$

and will decay with a time constant T_2^*, the spin–spin relaxation time modified by field inhomogeneity effects

$$\frac{1}{T_2^*} = \frac{1}{T_2} + \gamma \frac{\Delta \boldsymbol{B}_0}{2} \tag{2}$$

where $\Delta \boldsymbol{B}_0$ is the inhomogeneity of the main field.

Positional information necessary to form an image of the object can be obtained by applying magnetic field gradients during the evolution of the FID. The distribution of frequencies present in the FID will then be determined by the number of nuclei present at each position in the image field corresponding to a composite magnetic field made up of the static field and the field gradient. If the magnetic field gradients are linear, equation (1) becomes

$$\omega_x = \gamma \boldsymbol{B}_0 + \gamma x G_x$$

where ω_x is the NMR signal frequency at position x during the application of a field gradient G_x which introduces a linear variation of the Z field in the X direction. This equation embodies the basis of NMR imaging—the correspondence of signal frequency and position in a linear field gradient. Suitable selection of RF pulses prior to the data collection can produce an FID whose dependence on proton density (ρ), spin–lattice relaxation time (T_1) or spin–spin relaxation time (T_2) can vary. This will not be discussed in detail here since the principles of image reconstruction can be understood

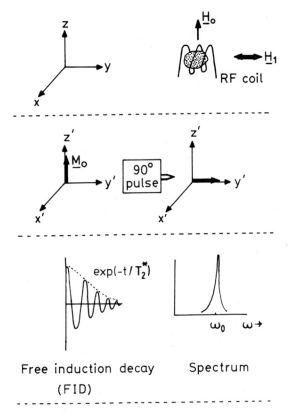

Figure 1. The basic NMR experiment.

from considering any FID signal and the influence of field gradients on it.

NMR imaging is an extremely flexible technique. A well designed imaging system will allow, within some technical limitations such as field gradient rise times or RF pulse powers, complete software-based control of radio-frequency pulse durations, frequencies and repetition rates, magnetic field gradient waveforms and timing in three orthogonal directions, and data sampling and collection. It is therefore possible for such a system to be used in a wide variety of different ways to scan the object and produce an NMR image. It is the purpose of this chapter to describe the basic principles of only the main variants of NMR scanning, since it is impossible to give an exhaustive account of all possible techniques. In particular, echo planar imaging[1] will not be discussed. Attention will be drawn to differences between methods in terms of signal-to-noise, scanning time and, where appropriate, computing time. Not all of the methods have been implemented in the present generation of clinical NMR scanners but continuing advances in computing may bring the more demanding ones within reach. In practical clinical imaging the scanning time is of great importance but must be weighed against the image signal-to-noise. NMR differs from x-ray computerized tomography in that the absence of biological hazard means that the scanning time may be freely increased to obtain signal to noise improvement.

4.2. Basic theory

It is not the purpose of this article to attempt to derive a relationship for the Free Induction Decay signal following a 90° pulse from basic NMR theory. The result in the case of generalized field gradients $G_x(t)$, $G_y(t)$, $G_z(t)$ is

$$S(t) = KM_0 \iiint_{x\,y\,z} \rho(x, y, z)$$

$$\times \exp\left[i\gamma \int_0^t (xG_x(t') + yG_y(t') + zG_z(t'))dt' + i\gamma B_0\right]$$

$$\times \exp(-t/T_2^*)dxdydz \qquad (4)$$

where K is a constant dependent on the receiver coil design and the electronic apparatus (Mansfield and Morris[1]). If phase sensitive detection is used then only the envelope in the FID is detected and the equation becomes

$$S(t) = KM_0 \iiint_{x\,y\,z} \rho(x, y, z)$$

$$\times \exp\left[i\gamma \int_0^t (xG_x(t') + yG_y(t') + zG_z(t'))dt'\right]$$

$$\times \exp(-t/T_2^*)dxdydz \qquad (5)$$

Notice that in the absence of field gradients the signal reduces to

$$S(t) = KM_0 \iiint_{x\,y\,z} \rho(x, y, z)dxdydz \times \exp(-t/T_2^*) \qquad (6)$$

an exponential decay with time constant T_2^* whose initial amplitude depends on the integral of the spin density distribution over the receiver coil volume.

In the case of linear constant field gradient applied for time t and writing $\omega_x = \gamma x G_x$, $\omega_y = \gamma y G_y$ and $\omega_z = \gamma z G_z$, equation (5) can be written

$$S(t) = KM_0 \iiint_{x\,y\,z} \rho(x, y, z) \times \exp[i(\omega_x + \omega_y + \omega_z)t]$$
$$\times \exp(-t/T_2^*)dxdydz$$

$$(7)$$

Examining this equation it can be seen that it has the form of a Fourier transform: thus a Fourier transformation of the FID signal can yield the spin distribution. In general, the transform will be three dimensional and, in a sense, several of the imaging methods may be considered as being techniques of reducing this computation to fewer dimensions through the use of suitable field gradients. Notice that the function $\exp[-t/T_2^*]$ is always convolved on the recorded signal and it is clear that magnetic field inhomogeneity must not be allowed to reduce T_2^* to a level where the effect of the gradients is not dominant. This point will be returned to later.

All NMR imaging techniques can be understood in terms of the above basic equation—the FID is a time function, but due to the linear relationship between signal frequency and spatial position introduced through the use of linear field gradients, its Fourier transform can yield the spin distribution directly.

4.3. Imaging methods

The flexibility of NMR imaging means that it is possible to image points, lines, planes or entire volumes of the object of interest (figure 2). The first

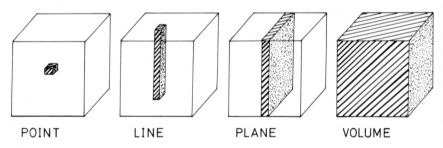

POINT   LINE   PLANE   VOLUME

Figure 2. Possible imaging techniques in NMR.

two of these possibilities are, at least for imaging systems, now probably of only historical interest since their signal to noise and scanning times are not suitable for practical clinical imaging. Imaging methods can be separated into two broad categories:

(1) Mapping methods which either build the image up through point or line scanning or calculate it directly with a multidimensional Fourier transform.

(2) Reconstruction methods which require, for example, a back projection operation to calculate the image from a series of projections which may either be line integrals or plane integrals.

The scan time, signal-to-noise ratio, resolution and computation time of the various varieties are all demonstrably different but experimental comparisons under well defined conditions have not been published.

4.4. Point scanning

Sensitive point scanning (Hinshaw[2]) is perhaps the simplest NMR imaging method and is based on the application of sinusoidal field gradients in the X, Y and Z directions with the object of defining a single point where the magnetic field is time invariant. All other points will experience complex time varying gradient fields. If the FID signal is passed through a low pass filter then the signal obtained is proportional to the spin density at that point. In the original experiments the frequency of the gradients was set at around 200 Hz for convenience and the sensitive point was moved by varying the phase shift between the waveforms.

In order to reduce the scanning time to reasonable levels the RF excitation was performed under conditions of steady state free precession (SSFP) where 90° pulses are applied sufficiently rapidly for an equilibrium magnetization to be set up. Nevertheless, the time required to image a single slice of the object to a resolution of 128×128 could still be around an hour. Additionally, the signal-to-noise ratio of the method is poor since the NMR signal is only received from a single "point" at a time and no averaging is carried out in the image formation.

4.5. Line scanning

The methods of line scanning that have been proposed (Mansfield *et al.*[3], Maudsley[4]) rely on the technique of selectively exciting only the nuclei in a slice of the object through the application of a field gradient during the RF pulse. Simplistically one can view this as depicted in figure 3; only nuclei in a volume where the magnetic field is appropriate for NMR frequencies within the bandwidth of the RF pulse will be excited. The slice shape is determined by the precise nature of the gradient and the RF pulse shape. The position of the slice within the object may be changed either by shifting the RF frequency or varying the amplitude of the field gradient. This technique is

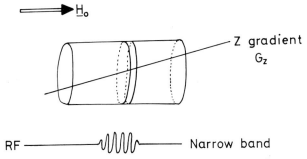

Figure 3. Slice selection by excitation during the application of a Z-gradient.

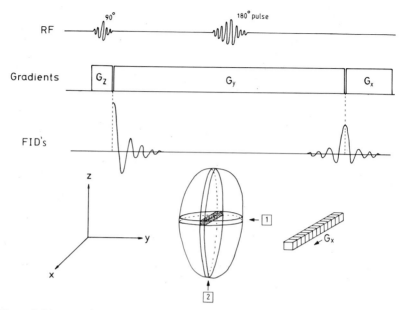

Figure 4. Line scanning through selective excitation of two planes and using an echo technique (Maudsley[4]).

used not only in line scanning but in all the imaging methods that deal with slices of the object. In the version of line scanning described by Maudsley a spin–echo technique is used (figure 4). Firstly a 90° RF pulse together with a G_z gradient selects a slice perpendicular to the z-axis. After a short time interval a 180° pulse together with a G_y gradient is used to select a further slice perpendicular to the first. The intersection of these two slices defines a line of voxels from which a spin echo is received after a time interval equal to the first. If a further G_x gradient is applied during the evolution of this spin echo, then from equation (5) the signal can be written

$$S(t) = KM_0 \exp(-\tau/T_2) \int \rho(x) \exp(i\gamma x G_x t) dx \qquad (8)$$

where τ is the time interval between the 90° and 180° pulses and the exponential factor including it allows for the use of a spin–echo technique. A 1-D Fourier transform of $S(t)$ will yield $\rho(x)$, the spin density along the selected line. As stated above, the position of the line can be varied by RF frequency or gradient amplitude adjustment and a whole slice can be mapped out to produce an image. Clearly, as in the case of point scanning, the signal-to-noise ratio will be a problem since a signal is only received from a line of voxels at one time.

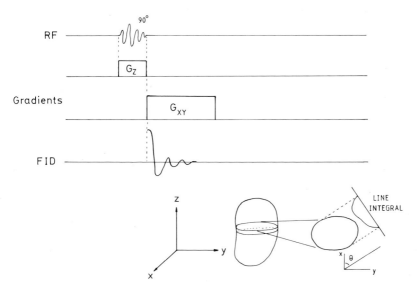

Figure 5. Two-dimensional slice scanning with reconstruction from line integrals.

4.6. Reconstruction methods

NMR imaging techniques that require a reconstruction of the image from projection data can be used in either 2-dimensional or 3-dimensional mode.

In 2-dimensional *slice scanning* (figure 5) a Z gradient is used at the time of RF excitation to excite selectively a single slice of the object. Gradients G_x and G_y are applied during the evolution of the FID signal and equation (5) reduces to

$$S(t) = KM_0 \iint_{x\,y} \rho(x, y) \times \exp[i\gamma(xG_x + yG_y)t]$$
$$\times \exp(-t/T_2^*)\mathrm{d}x\mathrm{d}y \qquad (9)$$

and writing $r = x\cos\theta + y\sin\theta$ where θ is the angle the composite gradient makes with the y-axis it can be shown that

$$S(t) = KM_0 \int_r I_1(r) \times \exp(i\gamma rG_r t) \times \exp(-t/T_2^*)\mathrm{d}r \qquad (10)$$

where $I_1(r)$ is a line integral of the spin distribution perpendicular to the applied composite G_r gradient. A 1-D Fourier transform of the FID signal will yield this line integral projection.

If a series of gradient combinations are used then the line integral projections can "rotate" round the object and a whole series of views are obtained. This situation is then entirely analogous to x-ray computerized tomography (Hounsfield[5]) and an image of the object can be reconstructed from this projection data by several well established mathematical techniques (Brooks and Di Chiro[6]); for example, back projection.

Figure 6 summarizes the operation. A Fourier transform of the collected FID yields the projection which must then be filtered before back projection. This may either be done through a convolution filter (Bracewell and Riddle[7]) or by multiplying the FID by a ramp prior to Fourier transformation, the latter being equivalent to the Ramachandran–Lakshiminarayanan[8] filter in x-ray computerized tomography. Computationally the back projection operation that follows is fairly demanding and requires either the use of microcode programming techniques or an array processor to achieve image reconstruction in a reasonable time.

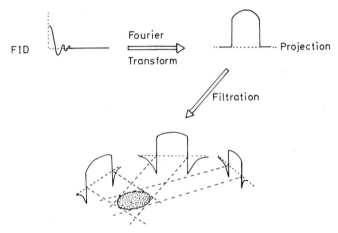

Figure 6. Backprojection reconstruction in NMR.

Fourier domain reconstruction (Mersereau and Oppenheim[15]) is also possible but is more conveniently discussed in detail in section 8 after direct Fourier methods have been dealt with.

Reconstruction from line integrals has several important signal-to-noise advantages in NMR imaging. Firstly, the signal is collected from an entire slice at once; secondly, the signal is collected directly after the 90° excitation pulse when it is at its largest; and, thirdly, if 180 projections (at 1 deg intervals) are used to reconstruct a 128 pixel square image then the image is over-determined and some signal-to-noise improvement occurs through averaging in the reconstruction process.

The disadvantages of back projection imaging are that image quality is very quickly degraded through inaccuracies in either the main static field or the gradient fields. Lai[9] has suggested that mathematically these two effects are separable and are capable of correction but this has not been experimentally demonstrated. Hounsfield (private communication) has proposed that automatic hardware correction for such effects is possible. If neither type of correction is attempted then the gradient non-linearity (ΔG) and main field inhomogeneity (ΔB) (both *absolute* values) must be exceeded by the absolute gradient strength in the following manner

$$G > \frac{(\Delta G + \Delta B)N}{L} \tag{11}$$

where N is the number of pixels across the image (typically 128) and L is the diameter of the image field. This condition is fairly stringent particularly if the static field is increased while attempting to keep the bandwidth constant (and hence the receiver Q).

Another problem with all methods that sample the FID directly after the application of field gradients is that it is not possible to switch the gradient on instantaneously and thus the initial part of the FID is not correct. Attempts to minimize this problem by using fast rise time gradients will produce problems caused by eddy currents generated in the magnet's metallic structure. Usually the initial sampling of the FID must be adjusted to allow for the gradient field settling. These essentially technical problems will not be discussed further but their presence does encourage the use of echo techniques.

Two dimensional slice scanning by back projection is not restricted to the examination of single slices during a scanning sequence. Since excitation is selectively restricted only to the slice chosen, and signal is only received from this set of nuclei, there is no reason why several separate slices cannot be excited one after the other (by frequency of Z gradient changes) and the signals from each of them collected one after the other. In this way excitations and data collections can be interlaced in the scanning period to make more efficient use of the available time. Each slice is still allowed several T_1 to relax between separate excitations but many slices can be dealt with during this time (figure 7). Multiple slice scanning sequences for up to thirty slices have been reported, the only disadvantage being that the resultant data rates require increased computer power, both in hardware and processing speed terms.

Although the description presented here has referred to slices at right angles to the Z-axis they can be in any orientation as long as the scanning equipment is capable of interchanging X, Y and Z gradients with equal sensitivities.

Scanning times per slice for back projection images are essentially given by a relationship like

$$T_S = N_\theta . t_R \tag{12}$$

where N_θ is the number of angles scanned (usually 180) and t_R is the repetition time of the sequence. Since several T_1 are required to allow the imaged material to relax completely T_S can be several minutes for a typical inversion recovery sequence with repetition time 1.4 s. Interleaving the slices is, of

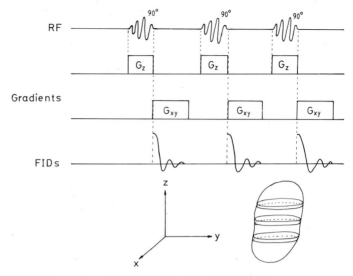

Figure 7. Multiple scanning with reconstruction from line integrals.

course, possible, so reducing the effective time per slice, although the whole set of slices still takes the same time.

At the time of writing it would appear that back projection reconstruction is being discarded in favour of direct Fourier methods (see next section) but its signal-to-noise advantages should be remembered.

Three dimensional reconstruction imaging does not use a selective excitation. Figure 8 illustrates the procedure in the case of using a Z gradient only during the evolution of the FID, and equation (5) reduces to

$$S(t) = KM_0 \int\limits_{z} \int\limits_{x} \int\limits_{y} \rho(x, y, z)\mathrm{d}x\mathrm{d}y \times \exp(\mathrm{i}\gamma z G_z t) \times \exp(-t/T_2^*)\mathrm{d}z$$

$$= KM_0 \int\limits_{z} I_p(z) \times \exp(\mathrm{i}\gamma z G_z t) \times \exp(-t/T_2^*)\mathrm{d}z \qquad (13)$$

where $I_p(z)$ is a plane integral perpendicular to the applied Z gradient. A 1-D Fourier transform of the FID will yield this plane integral. Clearly if a series of combination X, Y and Z gradients are applied then a series of plane integrals can be produced and a volume back projection can yield a volume image. Mathematically, the volume back projection is difficult and computationally demanding (Shepp[10]), in particular the computer must have a large memory. For a 128 point cubic image the available memory must exceed 4 Mbytes. The other disadvantage of this type of volume scanning is that it is necessary to collect around 10,000 FIDs to calculate an appropriate number of plane integrals so that the volume image will be fully determined. The

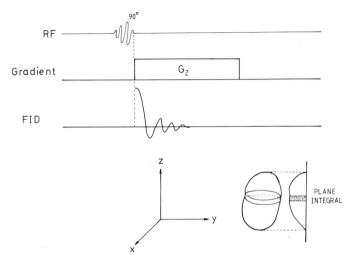

Figure 8. Excitation of an entire volume with reconstruction from plane integrals (Z gradient only shown).

resultant scanning time can easily approach an hour since the number of angles in equation (12) is now 10,000.

However, the attraction of constructing a volume image from which any desired plane may subsequently be selected is very strong, particularly when the effective thickness of each 2-D image is only one pixel. Such a thin slice width is not feasible in 2-D backprojection imaging since the signal-to-noise in that case is directly proportional to the slice width. In volume scanning the signal is collected from the entire volume simultaneously and signal to noise is very good.

At the time of writing, due to the prolonged scan time and the technical demands of collecting and processing such large amounts of data, 3-D back-projected images have not been widely demonstrated. Problems also exist in the RF bandwidth requirements and in the dynamic range of the FID signals.

4.7. Direct Fourier methods

Direct Fourier transform techniques were first proposed by Kumar, Welti and Ernst[11]. It is rather difficult to understand their mode of operation physically, but a mathematical formulation can be made quite simply. Recalling the usual form of the FID relationship for linear constant field gradients, G_x, G_y, G_z

$$S(t) = KM_0 \int\limits_x \int\limits_y \int\limits_z \rho(x, y, z)$$

$$\times \exp[i\gamma(xG_xt + yG_yt + zG_zt)]\,dxdydz \times \exp(-t/T_2^*)$$

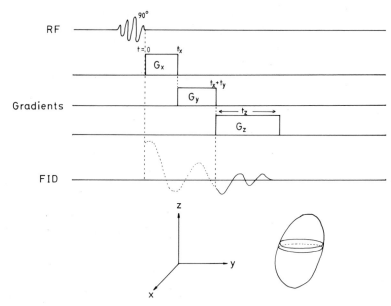

Figure 9. Excitation of an entire volume with reconstruction by direct Fourier technique.

The original formulation of 3-D direct Fourier imaging is illustrated in figure 9. A constant x gradient is applied for a time t_x followed by a y gradient for a time t_y and the FID is sampled during a time t_z in which a gradient G_z is applied. Variation of the times t_x and t_y at successive excitations can yield a set of signals

$$S(t_x, t_y, t_z) = KM_0 \int\limits_x \int\limits_y \int\limits_z \rho(x, y, z)$$
$$\times \exp[i\gamma(xG_xt_x + yG_yt_y + zG_zt_z)]\mathrm{d}x\mathrm{d}y\mathrm{d}z$$
$$\times \exp[-(t_x + t_y + t_z)/T_2^*] \qquad (14)$$

This procedure can be regarded as being suggested by the form of the equation above and clearly a 3-D Fourier transformation of the set of signals collected (represented by equation (14)) will yield the spin distribution $\rho(x, y, z)$.

The immediately apparent disadvantage of this method is that the signal is not sampled until after a time $t_x + t_y$ so that its amplitude will have significantly decreased due to spin–spin relaxation and its signal-to-noise will be degraded in comparison with methods that sample the FID immediately. This is particularly true for the larger values of t_x and t_y in the signal set. A more subtle point is that no averaging occurs in the image formation, unlike back projection methods where the image is generally over determined.

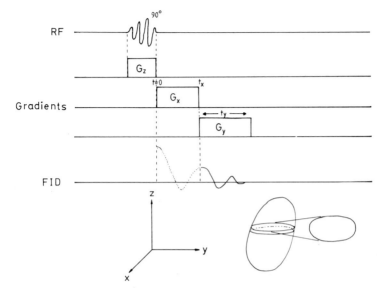

Figure 10. Two-dimensional slice scanning with reconstruction by direct Fourier technique.

Two-dimensional scanning is also, of course, possible by slice selection before application of successive gradients G_x and G_y during time periods t_x and t_y (figure 10). It is conventional to describe the first gradient as the phase encoding gradient.

Some of the disadvantages of this original formulation are removed in the spin–warp method (Edelstein *et al.*[12]) where the phase encoding gradient is kept on for a constant duration but its amplitude is varied in successive excitations (figure 11). From the form of equation (13) it can be imagined that the effect of this would be equivalent and in the next section this will be more clearly seen. This method tends to improve the signal-to-noise ratio and reduce the dependence on field homogeneity.

Computationally direct Fourier methods are straightforward and can be executed quickly. In 2-D imaging the row transforms can be done as scanning progresses but the column transforms must wait until scanning is over. Array processor hardware can perform the transforms very quickly and images can be available in a few seconds after scanning finishes. Again, with interchangeable gradients the imaged slice can be in any orientation and multislice imaging is possible through RF frequency or gradient variation. Scanning times can be slightly longer than the corresponding back projection image since for a 256×256 image 256 signals must be collected.

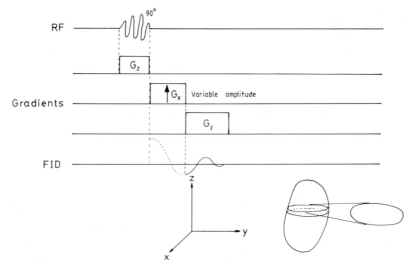

Figure 11. Two-dimensional slice scanning with reconstruction by direct Fourier technique. Alternative method utilizing a variation of the amplitude of the phase encoding gradient rather than its duration.

4.8. Comparison of methods

A convenient and elegant visualization and comparison of NMR imaging methods is possible through the k-space trajectory formulation of Ljunggren[13] and Twieg[14]. Suppose equation (5) is rewritten in vector form

$$S(t) = KM_0 \int \rho(r) \cdot \exp[i\gamma r \cdot \int_0^t G(t') dt'] dr \cdot \exp(-t/T_2^*) \qquad (15)$$

If the spatial frequency $k(t)$ is defined as

$$k(t) = \gamma \int_0^t G(t') dt' \qquad (16)$$

then

$$S(t) = KM_0 \int \rho(r) \cdot \exp(ik \cdot r) dr \cdot \exp(-t/T_2^*)$$

that is, the FID is simply a scaled representation of the Fourier transform of the object proton density distribution $\rho(r)$, a function of the spatial frequency distribution.

   The object of any NMR scanning procedure is to sample the k domain well enough for the spatial domain image to be retrieved from it (usually by means of a multidimensional Fourier transform). Sampling of the k domain is accomplished by sampling the FID, a time function, these processes being equivalent due to the correspondence of spatial position and signal frequency introduced through the use of field gradients.

The range of sampling of the k domain must include all spatial frequencies present in a significant amount in the object, and the frequency of sampling must match the size of the object.

Practical scanning methods for 2-D slices vary in the manner in which they map out the k_x, k_y plane. Figure 12 shows two examples. Projection

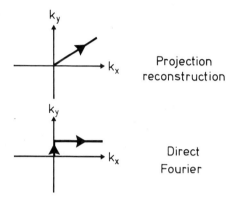

Figure 12. Scanning patterns in the k (spatial frequency) plane for projection reconstruction and direct Fourier technique.

reconstruction samples a series of radial lines depending on the relative values of G_x and G_y. Fourier imaging follows a path first up the k_y-axis (caused by the phase encoding gradient G_y) followed by a path along the direction of the k_x-axis through the G_x gradient. Clearly from the definition of k contained in equation (15) there is no difference between varying the time for which the phase encoding gradient is applied or its amplitude, since the integral and hence k can be the same. Subject to the constraints mentioned above, it is also possible to visualize the sampling of the FID required. Clearly in spin–warp imaging there is little point in successively sampling the region of excursion up the k_y-axis and, as mentioned earlier, only the k_x trajectory is sampled. The final result is a 2-D raster of k_x, k_y samples and a single 2-D FFT will produce the spatial domain image.

In projection reconstruction the final raster of k_x, k_y values is a polar one (figure 13) and image restoration is normally achieved by filtered backprojection. However, as discussed by Mersereau and Oppenheim[15] for x-ray CT, and by Jeong *et al.*[16] for NMR, it is also possible to calculate the corresponding cartesian raster through an interpolation scheme and then perform the normal 2-D FFT. In the x-ray case such a method is not very computationally efficient but in NMR, since the k space trajectories can be adjusted to minimize

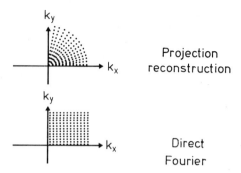

Figure 13. Sampling patterns in the *k* plane for projection reconstruction and direct Fourier technique.

the interpolation required, it is more attractive. The advantage over normal direct Fourier techniques is in terms of signal-to-noise ratio since the signal is sampled immediately after excitation.

Another useful feature of the *k* space description is that it is possible to visualize easily the formation of spin echoes. Any method that returns the trajectory to the origin results in the formation of an echo (e.g., figure 14(a)). This can either be accomplished by the application of an 180° RF pulse or through the reversal of the gradients. In figure 14(b) a possible gradient scheme to accomplish the scanning pattern of figure 14(a) is shown. Formation of several echoes is possible with the subsequent enhancement of signal to noise.

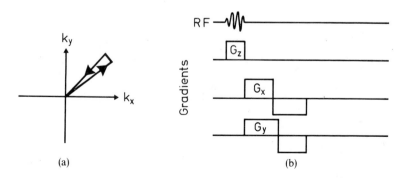

Figure 14. A gradient scheme (b) which samples *k* space as shown in (a) using spin echoes.

4.9. Conclusion

Nuclear magnetic resonance imaging has a unique flexibility since control of its scanning parameters is possible almost without constraint from a digital computer. Many questions remain to be answered regarding the optimal scanning schemes and future developments may lie in multiple echo schemes and three dimensional scanning.

References

1. Mansfield P and Morris P G 1982 *Advances in Magnetic Resonance, The Principles of Biological and Medical Imaging by NMR* (New York: Academic Press)
2. Hinshaw W 1976 Image formation by nuclear magnetic resonance: the sensitive point method *Journal of Applied Physics* **47** 3709
3. Mansfield P, Maudsley A A and Baines T 1976 Fast scan proton density imaging by NMR *Journal of Physics E: Scientific Instruments* **9** 271–278
4. Maudsley A A 1980 Multiple line scanning in NMR tomography *Journal of Magnetic Resonance* **41** 112–126
5. Hounsfield G N 1973 Computerized transverse axial scanning (tomography) *British Journal of Radiology* **46** 1016–1022
6. Brooks R A and Di Chiro G 1976 Principles of computer assisted tomography (CAT) in radiographic and radioisotope imaging *Physics in Medicine and Biology* **21** 689–732
7. Bracewell R N and Riddle A C 1967 *Astrophysical Journal* **150** 427–434
8. Ramachandran G N and Lakshminarayanan A V 1971 *Proceedings of the National Academy of Science, USA* **68** 2236–2240
9. Lai C M 1983 Reconstructing NMR images from projections under inhomogeneous magnetic field and non-linear field gradients *Physics in Medicine and Biology* **28** 925–938
10. Shepp L 1980 Computerized tomography and nuclear magnetic resonance *Journal of Computer Assisted Tomography* **4** 94
11. Kumar A, Welti D and Ernst R 1975 NMR Fourier zeugmatography *Journal of Magnetic Resonance* **18** 69
12. Edelstein W A, Hutchison J M S, Johnson G and Redpath T 1980 Spin warp NMR imaging and applications to human whole-body imaging *Physics in Medicine and Biology* **25** 751–756
13. Ljunggren S 1983 A simple graphical representation of Fourier-based imaging methods *Journal of Magnetic Resonance* **54** 338–343
14. Twieg D B 1983 The *k*-trajectory formulation of the NMR imaging process with applications in analysis and synthesis of imaging methods *Medical Physics* **10** 610–621
15. Mersereau R M and Oppenheim A V 1974 Digital reconstruction of multidimensional signals from their projections *Proceedings of the IEEE* **62** 1319–1338
16. Jeong J C, Song H B and Cho Z H 1982 Direct Fourier transform 3D image reconstruction with modified concentric square sampling—Application to NMR tomography. In *Proceedings of Meeting: Development of Multidimensional Image Processing Algorithms and Imaging Systems. Korea Advanced Institute of Science, Seoul, Korea, 1982*

CHAPTER 5 **The Aberdeen proton NMR imaging programme with primary emphasis on relaxation time**

J R Mallard

Department of Bio-Medical Physics and Bio-Engineering,
University of Aberdeen, Foresterhill,
Aberdeen AB9 2ZD, Scotland

5.1. Introduction

We now stand on the threshold of a completely new method of imaging, called nuclear magnetic resonance imaging or, in its more common abbreviated form, NMR imaging. In it, the protons of hydrogen in water and fat are located and imaged.

The protons of hydrogen behave like very tiny bar magnets of a definite strength, or magnetic moment. If they are placed in a magnetic field they will tend to line up more or less parallel to that field and will precess around it just like the spinning top does around the vertical gravitational field. The rate, or frequency, of this precession is proportional to the magnetic field strength in which they are placed.

By beaming on to them electromagnetic radiation of exactly the same frequency as their precession they absorb energy from the beam, which changes their alignment relative to the applied magnetic field. It is possible to turn them through 90° or through 180° at the time the magnetic field and the appropriate radiation are applied simultaneously. The frequency of radiation which has to be used is in the radiofrequency band, normally in the region of MHz or tens of MHz.

When the irradiating frequency is switched off, the excited nuclei have surplus energy which they radiate to their surroundings at the same resonant frequency. From a sample containing a large number of such nuclei, one by one they are then able to fall back, or relax, to their original alignment so that the sample re-emits its resonant frequency as a signal which can be detected and measured. The strength or intensity of the signal is proportional to the number of protons which relax per unit time, which is initially related to the number of protons present in the sample. Now the signal intensity will fall with time as more and more of the excited protons have relaxed. The length of time needed for this relaxation is associated with the environment of the protons—a measurement known as the relaxation time.

It helps to understand the principle of imaging using NMR by taking the simple example of two tubes of water lying side by side in a uniform magnetic field (figure 1). It is not possible to distinguish between the two tubes of water because both have been subject to the same magnetic field

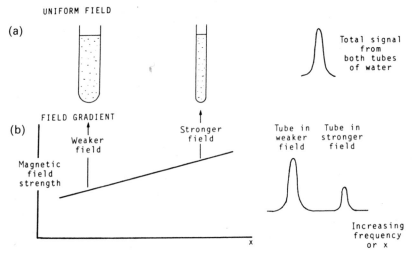

Figure 1. NMR spectra from test tubes of water: (a) uniform field, (b) field gradient applied.

and hence have the same resonant frequency; but if one now adds a field gradient to the applied magnetic field so that the field is stronger on one side than the other, one tube will now be in a slightly stronger field than the other and will resonate at a slightly higher frequency. The tube positioned in the higher field will absorb energy, and then re-emit it at a higher frequency than the other tube.

The use of a magnetic field gradient inside an NMR spectrometer makes it possible to identify position from the frequency of the emitted signal, the amount of water (or proton concentration) at a given position from the size of the signal from that position, and the relaxation time from the decay of that signal.

In the method which has been developed in Aberdeen since 1972, and which produced high quality clinical images in the summer of 1980, two images are built up to show the distribution of proton concentration, and of the longitudinal relaxation time (T_1), from a transverse cross-section of the body. The radiofrequency used in this Mk I machine is 1.7 MHz and the patient is placed in a magnetic field of 400 gauss (0.04 T), which is applied in the posterior–anterior direction of a supine patient.

The imaging principle employed is that of "selective excitation"[1, 2]. The particular form used (a form of two-dimensional Fourier transform called spin-warp imaging[3, 4, 5]) tolerates a much larger magnetic field non-uniformity than the projection reconstruction method[6, 7] and also the effect of patient movement is less drastic.

A 256 s scan collects data for both a proton density and T_1 image. The

T_1 value for each imaging element is calculated from the signal for the element without a $180°$ inversion pulse and the signal after one using a 200 ms relaxation time; the 128×128 element arrays are then interpolated into 256×256 arrays and displayed using 16 colour-coded levels, or grey scale.

The tomographic sections have a Gaussian profile with thickness (equivalent rectangular width) 18.5 mm. Each imaging element is 3.75 mm wide $\times$ 3.75 mm high $\times$ 18.5 mm thick, comprising a volume of about 0.26 cm^3. In each imaging element, the uncertainty in proton density for muscle tissue is about $\pm 2.5\%$, and the uncertainty in T_1 is about $\pm 3.5\%$ for T_1 close to 200 ms, with some worsening as T_1 departs from that optimum value.

The apparatus is described in detail in Hutchison *et al.* (1980)[8] and has resulted from the work of a team of people in this Department.

Of the human images shown in the lecture most were obtained with the NMR imaging method described above in the Mk I machine, a photograph of which is shown in Mallard (1981)[9]. A Mk II machine has been completed at the time of writing, using the same basic layout and imaging technique, but having improved signal-to-noise ratio, (more than twice) improved spatial resolving power, and improved patient ingress and egress and providing coronal and sagittal section views in addition to the transverse sections. This machine is the prototype of two models for commercial production* with a magnetic field strength of 800 gauss (0.08 T, 3.4 MHz).

To date, over 1500 patients and healthy volunteers have been examined using the technique and no short or medium term ill-effects have been experienced by or observed in any of the subjects[17].

Of the two available proton measurements, T_1 and proton density, each contributes valuable information about the anatomy and pathology seen on each section. Because T_1 values are dependent on the degree of water binding to tissue protein, they are the most valuable in characterizing soft tissue. Tissues such as muscle and liver, which have much protein-bound water, have short T_1 values (table 1) whilst other tissues such as cardiac muscle or spleen have longer values. Body fluids such as urine and cerebrospinal fluid (CSF) have long values. Whilst there is some overlap in the T_1 values of some normal tissues, their anatomical sites make identification simple and precise.

When malignant tissue is present it tends to have a T_1 value that is longer, from 25% to more than 100% longer, than the normal tissue in which it is situated, making for easy recognition of soft tumours[14]. Similarly, inflammatory and oedematous conditions are easily recognized and characterized. Table 2 summarizes T_1 values for normal and diseased states for tissue of the liver, averaged from *in vivo* measurements on patients using the Aberdeen Mk I NMR Imager using the colour coding and/or the region-of-interest programme. Table 3 gives data obtained in the same manner for brain pathologies. T_1 values measured at different magnetic field strengths and

*M & D Technology Ltd, Unit 1, Mastrick Industrial Estate, Aberdeen, Scotland.
Asahi Chemical Industry Ltd, Tokyo, Japan.

Table 1. Some typical spin–lattice relaxation times of human tissues. Measured from *in vivo* NMR images at 1.7 MHz

Tissue	Relaxation time (ms)
Normal	
Liver	140–170
Skeletal muscle	180–200
Bone	190–220
Eye	240–260
Cerebral cortex	250–300
Bile ducts	250–350
Kidney medulla	300–320
Kidney cortex	320–340
Blood	340–370
CSF	400–450
Fat	160–180
Pancreas	180–200
Cardiac muscle	240–260
Spleen	250–290
Cerebellar cortex	250–300
Spinal cord	290–300
Bile in gall bladder (depending on obstruction or not)	300–700
Urine	> 1000
Pathological	
Cirrhosis	180–300
Liver tumours	300–450
Lung carcinoma	350–400
Renal carcinoma	400–450

Table 2. T_1 values for liver, measured from *in vivo* NMR imaging at 1.7 MHz

	T_1 (ms)
Normal liver	140–170
Chronic active hepatitis	170–180
Cirrhosis	180–300
Secondary liver tumour	280–450
Hepatoma	300–450
Cholangiocarcinoma	200–350
Simple serous cyst	800–1000
Haemangioma	350–370
Ascitic fluid	700–1000

Table 3. T_1 values for brain, measured from *in vivo* NMR images at 1.7 MHz

		T_1 (ms)
Cerebrum	Grey matter	275
	White matter	225
Cerebellum		230–280
CSF		350–1000
Blood		340–370
Oedema		360–420
Haematoma		400–450
Infarct		320–375
Glioma		200–350
Meningioma		200–350
Metastases		200–350

frequency will not be the same as these values, but the relationship of T_1 values for two tissues at different frequencies will be similar. It is important to realize that the T_1 value measured *in vivo* for each pixel is a spatial average of a vast number of microscopic events over the volume of tissue in the pixel, and also a temporal average of all the microscopic events taking place during the period of data acquisition. Our understanding of relaxation phenomena is not fully established, but an excellent review is given by Foster[18].

The proton density images give a display of the proton concentration, which, in soft tissue, appears not to vary significantly from tissue to tissue, making the differentiation of soft tissue organs difficult on these images. However, there are significant differences in proton density between bone, soft tissue and fluids, and air, this fact enabling the easy recognition of bone and fluids when they are bounded by soft tissue. Fat is also easy to recognize. The proton density images are more akin to x-ray CT images.

The Aberdeen method (spin–warp) is tolerant of small body movements, both voluntary and involuntary, such as respiratory, cardiac and peristaltic motions, from which only small imaging artefacts arise. Also, there are no artefacts caused by gas/soft-tissue interfaces, nor by bone/soft-tissue interfaces, both of which can be troublesome on x-ray CT images. Also, the Aberdeen configuration of magnetic fields makes the images far less dependent upon the magnetic environment of the imager, and itself causes much less effect upon that environment. It also enables a more efficient radiofrequency system to be used which gives a very large gain in signal-to-noise ratio at the frequencies used. As a result, the quality of the images is similar to those obtained at more than twice the magnetic field strength, i.e., the 800 G Aberdeen images can compare well with those obtained from 2 kG field using superconducting magnets. The machine is light compared with others (1.5 tons) and installation and running problems and costs are far less. The advantages of the Aberdeen system are summarized in table 4.

This presentation was illustrated with human *in vivo* images of 30 patients

Table 4. Features of the Aberdeen NMR Imager

1. Measures T_1 and proton density section images simultaneously in 4.25 min.
2. Transverse, coronal and sagittal sections.
3. T_1 measured for each pixel provides:
   (a) True tissue identification
   (b) Maximum pathological contrast
   (c) Many lesions uniquely identified
   (d) Biochemical, physiological and anatomical measurements.
4. Aberdeen spin–warp method makes:
   (a) Images less spoiled by body movement.
   (b) Magnetic field need not be so uniform as others.
5. Unique configuration of vertical field makes:
   (a) Low magnetic field provide images equivalent to much higher magnetic field.
   (b) Resistive magnet give images as good as many superconductive magnet systems.
   (c) Installation and use easier.
   (d) Minimum exposure of patient to fields.
6. Vertical resistive magnet:
   (a) Reduces fringe field effects to surrounding equipment
   (b) Reduces effect on image from iron in building and surroundings
   (c) Makes projectile accidents unimportant.

selected from the Mk I clinical series [10–16] and some of the Mk II clinical series, from which figures 2, 3, 4, 5, and 6 are shown here.

It is clear that proton NMR imaging is a new but very important contribution to medical imaging, not only for diagnostic imaging of lesions and response to therapy, but also for systemic disease. In addition, it is a new, non-invasive tool to study physiological and biochemical phenomena *in vivo*, which will lead to a better understanding of living processes.

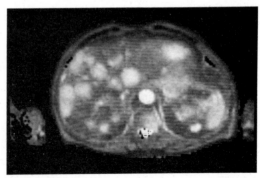

Figure 2. T_1 transverse image of secondary tumours in the liver from carcinoma prostate. The lumbar artery is also seen clearly.

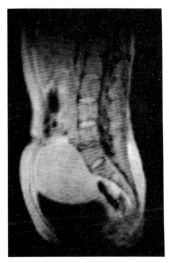

Figure 3. Proton density sagittal image of a large carcinoma of the ovary together with a prolapsed disc of the spine.

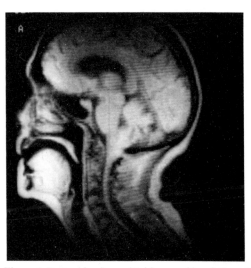

Figure 4. Proton density sagittal image of herniation of the cerebellar tonsils.

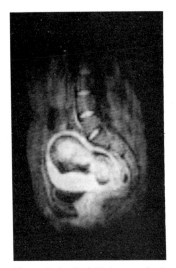

Figure 5. Sagittal D image of 16 weeks fetus before therapeutic abortion (D images contain both T_1 and proton density information).

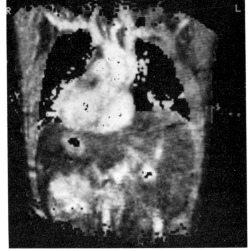

Figure 6. Coronal T_1 image of normal trunk showing heart and major blood vessels, liver, aorta, spleen.

References

1. Hutchison J M S 1976 Imaging by nuclear magnetic resonance. In Proc. 7th L. H. Gray Conf. *Medical Images* (Bristol Inst. of Physics and Wiley) pp. 135–141.
2. Mansfield P, Maudsley A A and Raines T 1976 Fast scan proton density imaging by NMR *Journal of Physics E: Scientific Instruments* **9** 271–278
3. Edelstein W A, Hutchison J M S, Johnson G and Redpath T 1980 Spin–warp NMR imaging and applications to whole-body imaging *Physics in Medicine Biology* **25** 751–756
4. Hutchison J M S, Sutherland R J and Mallard J R 1978 NMR Imaging; image recovery under magnetic fields with large non-uniformities *Journal of Physics E: Scientific Instruments* **11** 217–221
5. Sutherland R J and Hutchison J M S 1978 Three-dimensional NMR imaging using selective excitation *Journal of Physics E: Scientific Instruments* **11** 79–83
6. Ernst R R 1978 *Gyromagnetic resonance Fourier transform Zeugmatography* US Patent 4070, 611
7. Kumar A, Welti D and Ernst R R 1975 NMR Fourier Zeumagtography *Journal of Magnetic Resonance* **18** 68
8. Hutchison J M S, Edelstein W A and Johnson G 1980 A whole-body NMR imaging machine. *Journal of Physics E: Scientific Instruments* **13** 947–955.
9. Mallard J R 1981 The noes have it. Do they? Silvanus Thompson Memorial Lecture *British Journal of Radiology* **54** 831–849
10. Mallard J R, Hutchison J M S, Foster M A, Edelstein W A, Ling C R, Smith F W, Reid A, Selbie R, Johnson G and Redpath T 1981 Medical Imaging by Nuclear Magnetic Resonance; a review of the Aberdeen physical and biological programme *Medical Radionuclide Imaging 1980* (Vienna: IAEA) Vol. I, pp. 117–144
11. Smith F W, Mallard J R, Hutchison J M S, Reid A, Johnson G, Redpath T and Selbie R 1981 Clinical application of nuclear magnetic resonance *Lancet* **i** 78–79
12. Smith F W, Hutchison J M S, Mallard J R, Johnson G, Redpath T, Selbie R, Reid A and Smith C C 1981 Oesophageal carcinoma demonstrated by whole-body nuclear magnetic imaging. *British Medical Journal* **282** 510–512
13. Smith F W, Hutchison J M S, Mallard J R, Reid A, Johnson G, Redpath T W and Selbie R 1981 Renal cyst or tumour differentiation by whole-body nuclear magnetic resonance imaging *Diagnostic Imaging* **50** 61–65
14. Smith F W, Mallard J R, Reid A and Hutchison J M S 1981 Nuclear magnetic resonance tomographic imaging in liver disease *Lancet* **i** 963–966
15. Smith F W, Reid A, Hutchison J M S and Mallard J R 1981 NMR Tomographic Imaging—a new look at the pancreas *Radiology* **142** 677–680
16. Besson J A C, Glen A I M, Foreman E I, MacDonald A, Smith F W, Hutchison J M S, Mallard J R and Ashcroft G W 1981 Nuclear magnetic resonance observations in alcoholic cerebral disorder and the role of Vasopressin *Lancet* (October 24) 923–924
17. Reid A, Smith F W and Hutchison J M S 1982 Nuclear Magnetic Resonance Imaging and its implications: follow-up of 181 patients *British Journal of Radiology* **55** 784–786
18. Foster M A 1983 *Magnetic Resonance in Medicine and Biology* (Oxford: Pergamon Press)

CHAPTER 6 **Proton NMR imaging in clinical practice**

G M Bydder

Department of Diagnostic Radiology,
Royal Postgraduate Medical School,
Hammersmith Hospital, Du Cane Road,
London W12 0HS, England

6.1. Introduction

Since the first publication of NMR images of disease in the brain by Hawkes
et al. in 1980[1] many groups have begun programmes of clinical evaluation
and the results of these studies are now becoming available[2-4].

For a variety of reasons the brain has been the principal area of interest
in clinical NMR imaging. A high level of contrast is seen between grey and
white matter, providing excellent anatomical detail and a series of grey/white
matter interfaces for assessing mass effects. This high level of contrast also
enables the physiological process of myelination to be visualised in infancy
for the first time. Unlike x-ray computed tomography (CT) dense bone is
not a source of artefact. This is particularly important in the assessment of
the posterior fossa. Imaging is readily available in transverse, coronal, and
sagittal planes and there are a variety of sequences available, some of which
highlight blood flow and others of which highlight pathological changes.

Over a broad spectrum of neurological disease NMR imaging has proved
sensitive to pathological change. When this is coupled to the lack of known
hazard associated with the technique, a strong case can now be made for
the more general use of NMR in neurological practice. Experience in the
abdomen and pelvis remains limited but the early results are promising and
it is possible that NMR may come to play a useful role in imaging disease
within these regions of the body.

6.2. Technique

A variety of pulse sequences have been used with varying dependence on
proton density (ρ), T_1 and T_2 (table 1). Image interpretation has largely
proceeded on an empirical basis. Increases in T_1 and T_2 are seen in a variety
of pathological processes in which the water content of the lesion is increased,
e.g., inflammation, oedema, and many tumours, whilst a relative decrease in
T_1 is seen in such conditions as acute haemorrhage, fatty lesions, fibrosis,
and pleural thickening. The change in T_1 or T_2 may be 200–300% but is
relatively non-specific. Specificity is usually derived from localization and
the clinical context.

Table 1. NMR pulse sequences

Pulse sequence	Duration of scan cycle (ms)	τ (ms)
Saturation-recovery		
SR_{1000}	1000	
SR_{200}	200	
Inversion-recovery		
$IR_{1400/400}$	1400	400
Spin–echo		
$SE_{1040/20}$	1040	20
$SE_{1080/40}$	1080	40

6.3. Instrumentation and image interpretation

All NMR machines are constructed around a large magnet that provides a static magnetic field, B_0. In the presence of this field, hydrogen nuclei behave like tiny bar magnets. These are aligned with the static field resulting in a net proton magnetization M_0, in the direction of B_0.

A variety of sequences of radiofrequency pulses of different strengths are used to influence the magnetization and produce images with varying dependence on T_1 and T_2. Among the most useful of these are the saturation–recovery (SR) sequence which produces images whose contrast depends on changes in proton density (ρ), inversion–recovery (IR) whose contrast largely reflects changes in T_1, and spin–echo (SE) whose contrast reflects changes in both T_1 and T_2.

Another factor that affects the appearance of NMR images is the presence of flow and diffusion. The appearance of flowing blood, for example, depends on a variety of factors; the basic pulse sequence, the direction of blood flow, the slice selection technique, the relaxation time of blood, the use of cardiac gating, the use of spin-echo sequences for data collection, and other factors.

In spite of the multiparametric nature of the image, empirical rules have evolved permitting the choice of generally appropriate sequences. For example, in many disease states the change in proton density is relatively small (of the order of 10%) whilst the change in T_1 and T_2 may be several hundred per cent. In many diseases T_1 and T_2 are both increased so that disease may be recognized on inversion–recovery images as an increase in T_1 (which produces a dark appearance), and on spin–echo images as an increase in T_2 (which produces a light appearance).

6.4. Appearances of various conditions

There is now good agreement between different groups about the appearances of many common pathological entities [5–12] and some of this information is summarized below.

6.4.1. *Vascular disease*

Cerebral infarction results in a loss of grey/white matter contrast and an increase in T_1 on IR images. It also results in an increase in T_2. Infarction over the external surface of the brain and in the posterior fossa is generally better seen with NMR than with CT because of the absence of artefact and partial volume effects from bone. It is possible that changes in infarction may be seen earlier with NMR than with CT.

Acute haemorrhage produces a short T_1 similar to that of white matter on IR images and a normal or increased T_2 on SE images. Subdural haemorrhage is well demonstrated and it appears unlikely that problems will arise in the detection of "isodense" haematomas in the way that it has done with x-ray CT (figure 1).

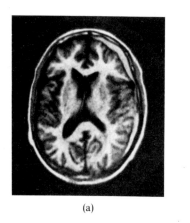 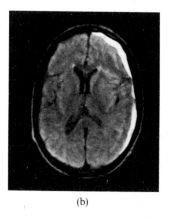

(a) (b)

Figure 1. Subdural haematoma: inversion-recovery (a) and spin–echo (b) scans. The haematoma has a short T_1 and appears light in (a). The haematoma has an increased T_2 producing a light appearance in (b).

Arteriovenous malformations and aneurysms have been identified because of their mass effects. Occlusion of vessels may be demonstrated by their failure to show highlighting of blood flow with rapid SR sequences.

6.4.2. *Cerebral infection*

Abscesses display the features of space-occupying lesions. Mass effects are well displayed with IR scans and the associated oedema is highlighted with SE sequences. Changes in herpes encephalitis are well seen in the temporal lobes.

6.4.3. Demyelinating disease

Following an early study comparing the results of contrast enhanced x-ray CT with NMR[13] several authors have confirmed the high sensitivity of NMR in detecting the plaques of multiple sclerosis (figure 2). In general, SE

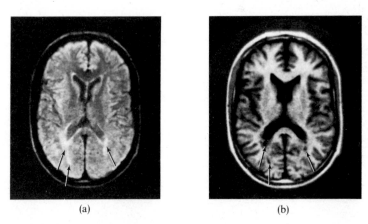

(a)   (b)

Figure 2. Multiple sclerosis: inversion–recovery (a) and spin–echo (b) scans. Lesions are seen on both scans (arrows).

sequences are more sensitive than IR sequences but there are exceptions to this rule. It is not clear whether the changes seen reflect the loss of myelin, the presence of oedema or a mixture of the two. Other demyelinating diseases such as the leucodystrophies (figure 3), central pontine myelinolysis and progressive multifocal leucoencephalopathy also show marked change. Abnormalities are readily seen in Binswanger's disease (subcortical arteriosclerotic dementia).

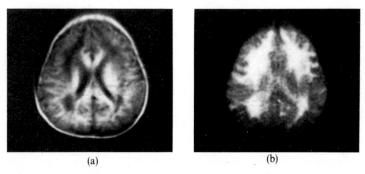

(a)   (b)

Figure 3. Leucodystrophy: inversion–recovery (a) and spin–echo (b) scans. The diffuse abnormality in the white matter is well demonstrated on both scans.

6.4.5. *Benign tumours*

Most tumours display an increase in T_1 and T_2 although there are exceptions. These are seen in lipid-containing tumours, in tumours that have undergone recent haemorrhage, and in other circumstances where the explanation is less clear.

Generally there is less oedema with benign than with malignant tumours. Meningiomas are clearly demonstrated. Acoustic neuromas are particularly well demonstrated. The dense petrous bones give little or no signal and this contrasts strikingly with the appearance of the normal facial and vestibulo-acoustic nerves in their intracannilicular course. It is thus possible to see small acoustic neuromas without the need for air or metrizamide enhanced CT.

A variety of other benign tumours have been shown and separation between intra- and extra-axial tumours within the posterior fossa is usually straightforward.

6.4.6. *Malignant tumours*

Although these tumours are early identified, separation between tumour and peritumoral oedema is not so easy (figure 4). In about 40% of cases this is much better shown with x-ray CT although stereotactic biopsy studies have confirmed the fact that tumour frequently extends outside the margin of enhancement shown with CT and that therefore the CT distinction between tumour and oedema can be spurious. Calcification within tumours is better shown with x-ray CT. As with other lesions NMR has a particular advantage in posterior fossa and foramen magnum tumours.

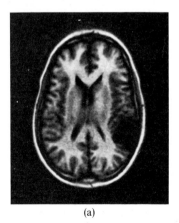
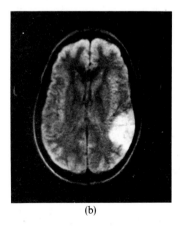

(a)   (b)

Figure 4. Astrocytoma Grade II: inversion–recovery (a) and spin–echo (b) scans. Although the abnormal area is well shown on both scans it is not possible to define the margin between tumour and oedema.

6.4.7. *Other diseases*

Cerebral and cerebellar degeneration are well displayed. The Arnold Chiari malformation lends itself to diagnosis with NMR using sagittal sections. Wilson's disease shows characteristic changes in the lentiform nuclei and basal ganglia. Hydrocephalus is well shown and oedema is seen at the ventricular margin in acute and subacute cases.

6.4.8. *Paediatric disease*

Not only can the normal phases of myelination be displayed, but delays in this process can be recognized. Previously, demonstration of delayed myelination was only possible at postmortem but it has now been recognized *in vivo* as a sequel to intraventricular haemorrhage and in cases of rubella infection and cerebral palsy.

The lack of known hazard is a particularly important consideration in children, where follow-up examinations may be required for a long period, in a variety of conditions such as hydrocephalus treated with ventriculoatrial shunts.

6.4.9. *The liver*

While it is possible to obtain satisfactory saturation–recovery images of the liver within breathholding times (e.g., 12.8 s), these images show a low level of contrast between normal and abnormal tissue. In routine practice it is therefore customary to use inversion–recovery and spin–echo images, which show superior contrast but require scan times of several minutes. These longer scan times (4–10 min) result in blurring of the image due to respiratory movement.

Saturation–recovery images of the liver are relatively featureless but blood flow in portal veins traversing the image slice may be highlighted. Inversion–

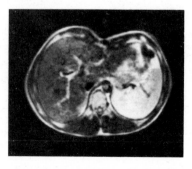

Figure 5. Normal liver: spin–echo scan. The portal vein appears light, the aorta is dark grey, and the inferior vena cava is black.

recovery images show the liver parenchyma appearing light (as a result of its short T_1) with blood vessels and bile ducts appearing dark. Spin–echo images show the liver parenchyma as darker. The appearance of blood flow with spin–echo images is variable depending on a variety of factors (figure 5).

Metastases are identified either by their dark appearance (due to an increase in T_1) on inversion–recovery images or as lighter areas on spin–echo images (due to an increase in T_2) (figure 6). It is frequently necessary to refer

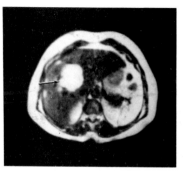

Figure 6. Liver metastasis: spin–echo image. The tumour appears light (arrow).

to more than one type of image to ensure that an apparent lesion is not simply a normal vascular structure. Several groups have reported accuracy of detection of metastases with NMR as similar to that of x-ray CT and ultrasound[14–16]. In four instances we have identified metastases not seen with x-ray CT. The lack of artefact from the air/fluid interface in the stomach is an advantage over CT in detecting metastases within the left lobe of the liver.

Primary tumours are also readily detected (figure 7) although the increase

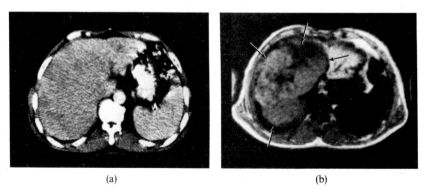

(a)   (b)

Figure 7. Hepatoma: contrast-enhanced CT (a) and inversion–recovery (b) scans. The tumour is poorly demonstrated in (a) but clearly demonstrated in (b) (arrows).

in T_1 and T_2 is generally less than that seen with metastases. The situation may also be complicated by the fact that many hepatomas occur in the liver of the patients with cirrhosis. Since both these diseases tend to produce an increase in relaxation times, contrast between the tumour and surrounding parenchyma may be small. Focal increases in T_1 and T_2 are also seen in benign tumours such as haemangiomas. Dilated bile ducts are readily recognized.

Liver abscesses are readily identified. Infective hepatitis also may result in an increase in T_1 although the changes are diffuse.

As mentioned previously cirrhosis may produce an increase in T_1 and T_2 although there is generally little change in the attenuation values of liver seen with x-ray CT. The normal T_1 value of the liver is only slightly greater than that of fat, and fatty infiltration results in little change of relaxation time.

Increasing iron content within the liver results in a decrease in T_1 and T_2 as a result of its paramagnetic effect. With a very large increase in iron the relaxation time of the liver may become so short that signal is no longer detectable in the liver, resulting in a dark appearances with all three groups of sequences. In a variety of other conditions the T_1 of the liver may be non-specifically increased. These include chronic active hepatitis and the Budd–Chiari syndrome.

6.4.10. *Gall bladder*

The gall bladder and biliary system are readily seen. In the fasting state layering is seen within the gall bladder as a result of the accumulation of bile salts and it has been suggested that this may form the basis for a test of biliary function[17].

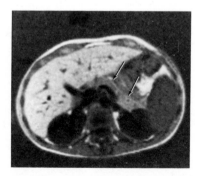

Figure 8. Normal pancreas: inversion–recovery scan. The normal pancreas (arrows) has a light appearance similar to that of the liver.

6.4.11. *Pancreas*

The normal pancreas has a relatively short T_1 and appears light on inversion-recovery images (figure 8). Large pancreatic tumours have been identified with NMR[18]. In one instance we have seen a pancreatic tumour which was not recognized with CT or ERCP.

Problems are experienced in distinguishing pancreatic tumours from the duodenum and other loops of bowel which normally have a long T_1 and T_2. There are also difficulties in distinguishing tumours from fat with the usual spin–echo sequences although it is possible to design pulse sequences that can do this. It is likely that oral contrast agents will be necessary in NMR in a way analogous to x-ray CT in order to circumvent the problem of distinguishing tumours from loops of bowel.

Acute pancreatitis and pseudocysts have also been identified in a similar way to x-ray CT. In four instances an increase in T_1 has been seen in chronic pancreatitis where no definite abnormality was seen with x-ray CT (figure 9).

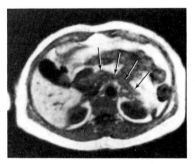

Figure 9. Chronic pancreatitis: inversion–recovery scan. The pancreas (arrows) appears dark compared with the normal pancreas shown in figure 8.

6.4.12. *The adrenal gland*

The normal adrenal gland can be seen without difficulty and hypertrophy, benign tumours, and metastases have been recognized[19].

6.4.13. *The kidney*

Inversion–recovery images are notable for the contrast between cortex and medulla which is apparent in the normal kidney (figure 10). In a variety of conditions, including acute and chronic glomerulonephritis, tuberculosis, and severe renal failure, this contrast is lost. Cysts and tumours are generally well seen, as is hydronephrosis.

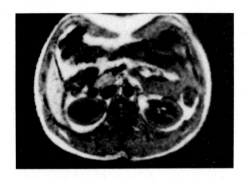

Figure 10. Normal kidneys: inversion–recovery scan. The distinction between cortex and medulla is readily seen.

The transplanted kidney is readily seen and the distinction between acute tubular necrosis and rejection has been made, although the role of NMR in relation to established techniques such as ultrasound, IVU and CT is yet to be determined.

6.4.14. *The retroperitoneum*

A variety of retroperitoneal tumours have been identified. Psoas abscesses have been seen and so have aneurysms of the abdominal aorta. Although enlarged lymph nodes are seen in a similar way to x-ray CT, whether or not infiltrated nodes can be distinguished from reactive hyperplasia is unresolved at the present time. Tumours have been identified in the prostate, ovaries and uterus.

6.5. Conclusion

Much more work remains to be done in the neurological field, yet the pattern of results and the general features of NMR imaging strongly suggest that this technique will come to occupy an important role in neurological diagnosis.

In some instances unique information is available from NMR imaging of the abdomen but ultrasound and CT also provide valuable information in a wide variety of disease. Many of the organs and tissues within the abdomen are accessible to biopsy, and a variety of other biochemical tests have specific roles in assessing disease within the abdomen and pelvis.

There are many current research developments such as flow imaging and the imaging of sodium-23 which have been demonstrated in the laboratory but have not yet been applied in clinical practice. It is also possible that respiratory gating may result in considerable improvement in image quality.

The use of paramagnetic contrast agents is another developing field. These agents, including molecular oxygen, iron, manganese and gadolinium, have the effect of decreasing T_1 and T_2. Gadolinium chelates have been used in animals and are being evaluated in humans. Not only do these materials act as contrast agents in their own right but they may be linked as markers to metabolites. antibodies and other compounds.

With improved technique direct measurements of T_1 and T_2 may prove to be of value although initial results seem to suggest that they are rather non-specific.

What role NMR will play in clinical practice remains to be seen but will certainly be the subject of intense interest over the next few years.

6.6. Acknowledgements

I am very grateful to Dr Ian Young and his team from Picker International and the General Electric Company who designed and built the NMR machine from which the above images were obtained.

References

1. Hawkes R C, Holland G N, Moore W S and Worthington B S 1980 Nuclear magnetic resonance (NMR) tomography of the brain: a preliminary clinical assessment with demonstration of pathology *Journal of Computer Assisted Tomography* **4** 577–586
2. Bydder G M, Steiner R E, Young I R, Hall A S, Thomas D J, Marshall J, Pallis C A and Legg N J 1982 Clinical NMR imaging of the brain: 140 cases *American Journal of Neuroradiology* **3** 459, and *American Journal of Roentgenology* **139** 215–236
3. Crooks L E, Mills C M, Davis P L, Brant-Zawadzki M, Hoenninger J, Aradawa M, Watts J and Kaufman L 1982 Visualization of cerebral and vascular abnormalities by NMR imaging: the effect of imaging parameters on contrast *Radiology* **144** 843–852
4. Johnson M A, Pennock J M, Bydder G M, Steiner R E, Thomas D J, Hayward R, Bryant D R T, Payne J A, Levene M I, Whitelaw A, Dubowitz L M S and Dubowitz V 1983 Clinical NMR imaging of the brain in children: normal and neurologic disease *American Journal of Neuroradiology* **4** 1013–1026
5. Mallad J 1981 The noes have it! Do they? *British Journal of Radiology* **54** 831–849
6. Luiten A L, Locher P R, Van Uijen C, Van Dijk P and Den Boef J 1982 Clinical results of NMR imaging. In *NMR Imaging* ed. R L Witcofski, N Karstaedt and C L Partain (Winston-Salem, NC: Bowman Gray School of Medicine) pp. 65–71
7. Bailes D R, Young I R, Thomas D J, Straughan K, Bydder G M and Steiner R E 1982 NMR imaging of the brain using spin-echo sequences *Clinical Radiology* **33** 395–414
8. Weinstein M A, Modic M T, Starnes D L, Pavlicek W, Gallagher J and Duchesneau P M 1982 Nuclear magnetic resonance: comparison on inversion-recovery, saturation-recovery and usefullness of T_1 measurements of the brain in tumours (abstract). Scientific program, *Society of Magnetic Resonance in Medicine* p 152 (Society of Magnetic Resonance, Boston).
9. Zeitler E and Schuierer G 1983 NMR clinical results: Nuremburg. *Nuclear Magnetic Resonance (NMR) Imaging* ed. C L Partain, A E James, R R Price and F D Rollo (Philadelphia: Saunders) pp. 207–230
10. Buonanno F S, Brady T J, Pykett I L, Burt C T, Vielma J, New P F J, Newhouse J H, Taveras J, Hinshaw W S, Goldman M R, Kistler J P and Pohost G M 1983 NMR clinical results: Massachusetts General Hospital. *Nuclear Magnetic Resonance (NMR) Imaging* ed. C L Partain, A E James, R R Price and F D Rollo (Philadelphia: Saunders) pp. 207–230
11. Huk W and Loeffler W 1983 NMR clinical results: Erlangen. *Nuclear Magnetic Resonance (NMR) Imaging* ed. C L Partain, A E James, R R Price and F D Rollo (Philadelphia: Saunders) pp. 276–294

12. Bydder G M, Steiner R E, Thomas D J, Marshall J, Gilderdale D J and Young I R 1983 NMR imaging of the posterior fossa: 50 cases *Clinical Radiology* **34** 173–178

13. Young I R, Hall A S, Pallis C A, Legg N J, Bydder G M and Steiner R E 1981 Nuclear magnetic resonance imaging of the brain in multiple sclerosis *Lancet* **ii** 1063–1066

14. Smith F W, Mallard J R, Reid A and Hutchison J M S 1981 Nuclear magnetic resonance tomographic imaging of liver disease *Lancet* **i** 963–966

15. Doyle F H, Pennock J M, Banks L M, McDonnell M J, Bydder G M, Steiner R E, Young I R, Clarke G J, Pasmore T and Gilderdale D J 1982 Nuclear magnetic resonance (NMR) imaging of the liver: initial experience *American Journal of Roentgenology* **138** 193–200

16. Margulis A R, Moss A A, Crooks L E and Kaufman L 1983 Nuclear magnetic resonance in the diagnosis of tumors of the liver *Seminars of Roentgenology* **18** 123–126

17. Hricak H, Filly R A, Margulis A R, Moon K L, Crooks L E, and Kaufman L 1983 Nuclear magnetic resonance imaging of the gall bladder *Radiology* **147** 481–484

18. Smith F W, Reid A, Hutchison J M S, and Mallard J R 1982 Nuclear magnetic resonance imaging of the pancreas *Radiology* **142** 677–680

19. Moon K L, Hricak H, Crooks L E, Gooding C A, Moss A A, Engelstod B L and Kaufman L 1983 Nuclear magnetic resonance of the adrenal gland: a preliminary report *Radiology* **147** 155–160

CHAPTER 7 **Clinical ^{31}P NMR spectroscopy**

E B Cady, D T Delpy and P S Tofts

University College Hospital,
London, England

7.1. Introduction

Prior to the development of NMR imaging (NMRI), NMR spectroscopy (NMRS) found its place in the analytical chemistry laboratory during the early 1950s. *In vivo* NMRS is a harmless and non-invasive method[1, 2, 3] for determining relative concentrations of metabolites and intracellular pH[4] and studying their relationship to pathology or induced biochemical change. The determination of absolute concentrations is difficult, mainly because the quantity of tissue sampled and the radio frequency (RF) absorption may only be evaluated in simple cases. An extensive literature exists describing the achievements of biological NMRS including both "test-tube" and *in vivo* results[5 − 10].

There are many basic texts to which the reader can turn for the relevant fundamentals of NMR[11 − 13]. The main difference between NMRI and NMRS is due to a different technical application of the theory. The basic relationship upon which all NMR depends is that the resonant frequency of the nuclear system is proportional to the "local" magnetic field strength (the constant of proportionality is called the gyromagnetic ratio and is related to the nuclear magnetic and angular moments). In NMRI the nucleus (usually the proton) is positionally labelled by its resonant frequency in a known magnetic field gradient. Only relatively coarse frequency resolution is required and signals from protons in all molecular species are detected together, although the H_2O signal predominates. Large field gradients are applied to the sample and due to the coarse frequency resolution only the applied field is relevant. For NMRS very homogeneous fields are used (usually uniform to one in 10^8 for analytical laboratory spectrometers, although magnets with bores wide enough to allow the insertion of human limbs are at present only capable of one in 10^7) and this means that the local magnetic fields produced by molecular electrons label the nuclei with resolvable resonant frequencies. Hence similar nuclei in molecular species with different electronic structures will resonate at different frequencies and a spectrum can be obtained allowing a chemical assay to be made. The frequency difference caused by this effect is termed the "chemical shift" (CS) and this is usually measured in units of parts per million (ppm) of the magnetic field rather than in hertz. This allows the immediate comparison of spectra obtained from different strength magnets. The ppm scale is defined relative to a reference resonance by the following relationship

$$CS = 10^6 \times (f_s - f_r)/f_r \text{ ppm} \tag{1}$$

where f_s is the shifted frequency and f_r is a reference resonance frequency adopted for a particular application.

Due to the dependence of resonant frequency on field strength, it follows that better resolution is obtained with strong magnets and those in use are typically about 2 to 10 T (1 T = 10^4 gauss). Only nuclei in mobile metabolites (i.e., in solution) produce narrow spectral lines. Non-mobile nuclei (e.g., phosphorus in bone) give very broad resonances which can be removed from the spectrum by computer processing. The integral of each resonance is proportional to the total number of nuclei in that particular molecular species and so relative concentrations can be measured.

The magnetic field homogeneity is corrected and checked before each investigation by a process known as "shimming". Most biological tissues contain so much water that it is possible to construct RF coils tuned to a particular nuclear species but also able to detect a strong ^1H signal. The RF response of the system to a short RF pulse decays with time and is called the free induction decay (FID). By monitoring this signal and slightly altering the magnetic field contributions from various ancillary resistive coils (shim coils) it is possible to optimize the field homogeneity[14, 15] so that adequate spectral resolution is obtained.

An important aspect of *in vivo* NMRS is the method by which the tissue sample is specified and surrounding tissues excluded so the spectrum is not contaminated with unwanted signal. There are several techniques for achieving this and often the approach adopted will incorporate a combination of methods. For the examination of patients usually a one or two turn, planar RF coil (a surface coil) is placed on the skin adjacent to the tissue of interest[8]. The coil is used for both pulse transmission and FID reception. The RF field of the coil defines a coil volume which is roughly a cylinder of equal diameter to the coil and extending a radius into the tissue. Simple phantom measurements can be made to determine the length of RF pulse required to maximize the signal at the surface. It is also possible to determine the pulse length required to minimize the surface signal and this provides a method for reducing unwanted signals from tissues close to the coil[16]. This approach is useful in ^{31}P NMRS studies of brain, kidney and liver etc. when it is necessary to exclude spectral contributions from subcutaneous muscle. A further development is "field profiling"[17, 18] in which ancillary resistive coils are used to superimpose a specially designed field onto the main field. The additional field has a roughly spherical homogeneous region with adjustable diameter at the magnet centre. Outside this region are large field gradients so narrow resonances are only detected from within the homogeneous volume. The broad resonances picked up from outside this region can be removed from the spectrum by a computer technique known as "profile correction"[18].

Because of the large water content of most tissues (about 40 molar) reasonable proton spectra can be obtained from the Fourier transform of a single FID. In the case of ^{31}P and ^{13}C it is necessary to sum many FIDs (usually more than 100) in order to obtain spectra with adequate signal-to-noise ratio (SNR). This is due to the lower tissue concentrations and intrinsic sensitivities of these particular nuclei. (The ^{31}P concentration in normal muscle is about 25 mmol and assuming a ^{13}C relative abundance of 1%, muscle containing 10% fat has 65 mmol ^{13}C.)

A phenomenon called "saturation" arises from the requirement for a period of nuclear relaxation before the arrival of the next RF pulse. This relaxation time is approximately $5T_1$ where T_1 is the spin–lattice relaxation time constant[19]. If the pulse interval is much less than this, satisfactory relaxation does not occur and the FID is smaller in amplitude. A problem posed by this and the necessity of adding several hundred sequentially acquired FIDs together is the determination of the pulse rate and pulse length giving maximum SNR for the total available acquisition time. (Patients, unlike test-tube samples, cannot be left sitting with a limb in a magnet for extended periods of time.) For a given number of pulses the SNR obtained will increase with the interval between pulses[19-21] but a given total acquisition time will contain fewer pulses if the intervals are longer and hence optimum pulse intervals and lengths have to be determined. The relaxation times for nuclei in various metabolites are different and this means that the amount of signal reduction caused by rapid pulsing will be dependent on metabolite. Although SNR may be improved by rapid pulsing (because more FIDs are acquired in a given time), measurements of metabolite concentrations will alter. To rectify this while still preserving the advantage of high SNR, "saturation factors" are applied to the measurements. These are determined from investigations on tissue using very long pulse intervals so that the relative spectral line integrals are directly related to concentrations.

The spectrometers used for *in vivo* NMRS are very similar to the systems available for conventional chemical analysis[22]. The only significant differences are at the "front end". Surface coils are used instead of solenoidal or saddle coils and additional profiling coils are incorporated to produce a controlled homogeneous volume. The main magnetic field used in clinical work has a horizontal axis as opposed to the conventional vertical configuration used in analytical laboratories. The horizontal field facilitates insertion of the patient but also means that a stronger field is experienced by magnetic floor objects (implying greater potential hazard).

Early NMR spectrometers were continuous wave instruments and samples were interrogated by frequency scanning. The introduction of pulsed NMR[21] and the analysis of FIDs by computerized Fourier transform techniques[21, 23] has greatly increased the flexibility available for data acquisition and analysis. A schematic diagram of a typical system for *in vivo* NMRS is shown in figure 1.

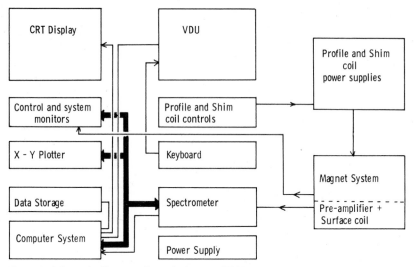

Figure 1. Schematic diagram of a typical *in vivo* NMR spectrometer system.

7.2. Radio frequency coils for NMR spectroscopy

7.2.1. Coil theory

(i) *Design criteria*

The front end of the spectrometer is shown in figure 2. The coil is resonated by a fixed capacitor C_f and a small variable capacitor C_t. Matching to the coaxial line is through a variable capacitor C_m. Crossed diodes prevent transmitter leakage from reaching the coil during the receive period. Attention to detail is necessary in order to achieve the best possible SNR. Our design criteria for the coil are that:

(1) The SNR should be maximized and the method can be derived from Hoult and Richards (1976)[24]:

$$\text{SNR} \propto V_s(Q/V_c)^{1/2} \tag{2}$$

where Q is the quality factor of the coil, V_c is the coil volume and V_s is the effective sample volume, i.e., the volume of sample within the coil volume.

To maximize SNR for a given sample volume, we need to:

(a) Maximize the Q of the coil when loaded by the sample. The sample is electrically conducting and this usually constitutes the major source of coil damping. The coil itself and its immediate surroundings should be constructed from materials with low dielectric loss.

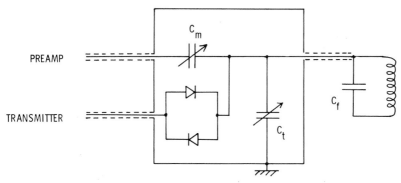

Figure 2. The coil match and tune circuit of the spectrometer "front end".

(b) Minimize the coil dimensions within the constraints of keeping the sample within the coil volume and of practical clinical considerations. This is a complex problem which requires a sophisticated understanding of the spatial response of the coil, how Q decreases as a greater proportion of the coil volume is filled with lossy sample and a detailed knowledge of the anatomy of the tissue. At present the only approach available is empirical and is based on measuring actual SNR for various geometries. The materials used near the coil should be non-ferrous, in order to avoid introducing inhomogeneities in B_0 (the static magnetic field.)

(2) If the coil is to be used inside ^1H imaging coils with pulsed gradients the amount of conductor must be minimized to avoid field distortions or heating.

Surface coils[8] have been used for all our clinical spectra—however other configurations are under investigation. The shape of the coil can be altered to increase the effective sample volume, for example, a planar coil has been given a slight curve in order to fit limbs.

(ii) Match and tune circuit

The coil is in close proximity to the patient in order to achieve a good effective sample volume. However the capacitance between coil and patient, and the patient conductivity, cause extra losses in the resonant circuit and reduce Q[25]. A spacer, consisting of PTFE sheet about 2 mm thick, or a Faraday screen[25] may be used to reduce this effect. A fixed capacitor on the coil C_f provides most of the capacitance; fine tuning is achieved with a small variable capacitor C_t. In order to maximize SNR the resonant circuit is noise-matched[21] through a second variable capacitor C_m to the 50 Ω line. The crossed diodes act as a switch preventing any leakage from the transmitter from reaching the coil or preamplifier. The process of tuning and matching can be carried out by connecting an RF bridge in place of the preamplifier, and adjusting C_t and C_m until the bridge measures 50 Ω looking at the matched coil. The matching conditions are:

$$4\pi^2 f^2 LC = 1 \tag{3}$$

and

$$C_m^2 = C/(2\pi f Q Z_1) \tag{4}$$

where f is the resonant frequency, L the coil inductance, C the total capacitance $(C = C_m + C_t + C_f)$ and Z_1 the line impedance (50 Ω in this case). This matching process must be repeated for each patient, because Q is different for each sample of tissue. Provided the matching capacitor has been calibrated (section 7.2.2(iii) below), values of Q can immediately be obtained. Q can also be measured directly (section 7.2.2(iv)) and the above expression has been verified experimentally for a range of coils. The matching circuit can be thought of as a transformer, with a voltage ratio of

$$\frac{v_c}{v_l} = \frac{1}{w\pi f C_m Z_1} \tag{5}$$

where v_c and v_l are the coil and line peak to peak voltages. For $C_m = 10$ pF this ratio is 9.8. The transmitter pulse is about 100 V peak to peak, so at least 1 kV peak to peak may be present on the coil.

(iii) Flip angle

For a plane circular coil the ^{31}P transmitter pulse length required to produce a given flip angle on axis can be derived. The flux at an axial distance x from the coil (radius a) is given by[26]

$$B_1 = \frac{\mu_0 n i}{2} \frac{a^2}{(a^2 + x^2)^{3/2}} \tag{6}$$

where i is the current, n the number of turns and μ_0 the permeability of free space $(4\pi \times 10^{-7}$ H m$^{-1})$. The current is given by

$$i = v_c/2\pi f L = v_1 C/Z_1 C_m \tag{7}$$

The flip angle θ for a pulse of length τ_θ is given by

$$\theta = \gamma B_1 \tau_\theta / 2 \tag{8}$$

where γ is the gyromagnetic ratio $(1.72 \times 10^7$ Hz T^{-1} for ^{31}P; 1.07×10^7 Hz T^{-1} for ^{13}C). The factor 2 arises because the linear field B_1 is resolved into two circular fields of amplitude $B_1/2$, one of which is static in the rotating frame[13]. Combining equations (6), (7) and (8) we have

$$\tau_\theta = \frac{4\theta Z_1 C_m a}{C v_1 \gamma \mu_0 n} \frac{(a^2 + x^2)^{3/2}}{a^3} \tag{9}$$

and experimentally measured values of 180° pulses are in broad agreement with this. The flip angle is proportional to C_m, so having found it for one sample we can calculate the length required for another sample of different dielectric loss provided that the geometry is similar.

(iv) Noise

Two sources of noise are relevant:
(1) Thermal noise: the RMS noise voltage v_n from a resistance R at temperature T is given by

$$v_n^2 = 4kT \, df R \qquad (10)$$

where df is the bandwidth. Since the coil has been matched to 50 Ω at the preamplifier input, it produces the same thermal noise as a 50 Ω resistor connected to the preamplifier input.
(2) RF pickup from a variety of sources such as radio transmitters, motors and switches.

The RMS noise at the receiver output can by monitored. By connecting a 50 Ω terminator the value of thermal noise can be measured—any extra noise is caused by RF pickup. Since the measurement time to achieve a given SNR is proportional to the square of the noise, it is important to minimize this interference.

7.2.2. Coil construction

(i) Materials

In order to use the same variable capacitors (1–20 pF) with all coils, the fixed capacitor should be in the range 100–250 pF. For a small coil diameter this means using several turns to obtain sufficient inductance. The capacitors must be chosen with care; they must be non-ferrous, withstand the large RF voltages, have a high Q and the fixed ones must be physically small to avoid unwanted lead inductance. For the latter we use ceramic thick film chip capacitors (American Technical Ceramics, 1 Norden Lane, Huntingdon Station, NY 11746, USA. UK agent ATC Capacitors Ltd, Crawley, Sussex) although standard silver mica capacitors are probably acceptable provided they are physically small. The variable capacitors are PTFE-dielectric tubular 4-turn 2.5 kV DC breakdown voltage (cat no. 4456, Jackson Brothers (London) Ltd, Croydon CR9 4DG, UK).

(ii) Selection of fixed capacitor

The procedure for selecting the fixed capacitor for a given coil is now described. The coil is connected to the tune and match network in the standard way. The RF bridge is used to drive a crude loop aerial, the radiation from which is picked up by the coil. This pickup is monitored using an oscilloscope connected to the preamplifier output. The approximate fixed capacitance needed to resonate the coil may be estimated by either of two methods:

(1) Temporarily connecting a large (500 pF) variable capacitor across the coil and observing the resonance as a peak in the preamplifier output.
(2) Using the formula[27] for the inductance of a plane circular coil

$$L = \mu_0 a n^2 [\ln(8a/b) - 2] \tag{11}$$

where b is the radius of the wire. The exact value can be found by observing the preamplifier output as the variable tuning capacitor is adjusted near to resonance.

(iii) Calibration of variable capacitor

The small variable capacitors may be calibrated as follows. Using a coil of the highest possible Q, the change in tuning capacitance (in turns) to produce a given change df in resonant frequency is measured. These are related through

$$dC = -2C \, df/f \tag{12}$$

where dC is the capacitance change. Care must be taken not to leave the flat portion of the preamplifier response curve and several measurements should be made to ensure dC is proportional to df.

(iv) Direct measurements of Q

The Q of a matched coil may be measured directly by observing the change in voltage output at fixed frequency as the variable tuning capacitor is moved through resonance:

$$v_c = [1 + (Q \, dC/2C_0)^2]^{-1/2} \tag{13}$$

where dC is the amount by which C has been changed from the resonance value C_0. If the capacitance between the 3dB points (v_c reduced by a factor 0.7) is $2dC_{3dB}$ and between the 6dB points (v_c reduced by a factor 0.5) is $2dC_{6dB}$ then two estimates of Q may be obtained:

$$Q = 4C_0/2C_{3dB} \tag{14}$$

$$Q = 4\sqrt{3}C_0/2dC_{6dB} \tag{15}$$

Care must be taken not to operate the preamplifier beyond the linear part of its response.

7.2.3. Coil performance

For convenience of positioning, the coils are often on flying leads (35 cm of double-screened silver-plated copper coaxial cable 100 pF m^{-1}, type RG223/U). Table 1 shows the smallest and largest coils that have been used. The 74 mm coil used for neonatal brain has a high Q when unloaded, but this comes down dramatically when loaded. The 12 mm coil used for rat brain is affected less severely because of its smaller size[28]. Table 2 shows relative RMS noise for a variety of configurations. Because the infant and rat configurations are almost completely screened by the magnet bore, they pick up little RF and the noise is very near the minimum attainable. Larger subjects act as aerials, particularly when lying down. The effect of this has been reduced by earthing the limb close to the coil. A reduction in measurement time could probably be achieved with a Faraday cage.

Table 1. Coil parameters

Coil diameter (mm)	Number of turns	C_f (pF)	Q (unloaded)	Q (loaded)
74	1	100	600	110
12	3	240	300	210

Table 2. Noise from various patient configurations

Noise source	Relative RMS noise	Relative measurement time
50 Ω terminator	1	—
Infant or rat	1	1
Sitting adult	1.5	2.25
Lying adult	2	4

7.2.4. Quality control

Three parameters are monitored.
   (1) *Matching capacitor.* Q can be monitored with the matching capacitor using equation (4) and calibrating the matching capacitor as described in section 7.2.2. (iii) above. This has enabled us to detect and eliminate some sources of loss, such as conducting fluid on the coil, whilst studying exposed rat scalp and a bad patient earth connection. The pulse length τ required to obtain a given flip angle depends on the sample losses (through Q); changes in sample losses may be compensated by keeping τ proportional to C_m (see equation (9)).
   (2) *Linewidth.* B_0 must be shimmed to obtain optimum homogeneity for each patient. The coil is double tuned[15] to the ^1H and ^{31}P resonance frequencies (80 and 32 MHz) thus producing sufficient ^1H SNR with

a single FID. It is important to ensure that the ^{1}H signal comes from the same volume of tissue as the ^{31}P signal by choosing the pulse length correctly. This may be done as follows. The ratio of ^{1}H pulse length to ^{31}P pulse length, for any given angle, is a constant dependent only on the coil, its loaded Q, and the connecting components. This ratio may be measured, most easily for a 180° pulse on a small sample at a given distance from the coil, when a null signal may be obtained. This ratio may then be used to scale any ^{31}P pulse length to find the ^{1}H pulse length that will produce the same flip angle. This approach ignores the variation of RF absorption with frequency; however the skin depth at 80 MHz is at least 10 cm[29] so for depths up to 3 cm we believe it is reasonable to ignore this effect as a first approximation.

(3) RMS noise. This is compared with previous values and the 50 Ω value, as a check on RF pickup.

7.3. Patient handling and monitoring

7.3.1. General considerations

At University College Hospital, NMRS is applied to two major clinical areas of interest. Firstly, the study of muscle metabolism in children and adults; secondly, the study of brain metabolism in premature and term infants. Each application presents its own particular difficulties associated with the handling of the patient, and the monitoring of necessary physiological variables while in the magnet. There are, however, several problems that are common to both applications. The major one is that of correctly positioning the tissue of interest with regard to the homogeneous magnetic volume (if used) and the surface coil. The problem is illustrated in figure 3. The magnetic homogeneous volume is an approximately spherical volume on the magnetic axis.

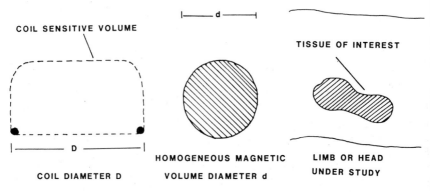

Figure 3. Schematic representation of the volume interrogated by a surface coil, the homogeneous magnetic volume and the tissue volume to be studied.

The diameter can be adjusted from 14 to 40 mm or can be switched off if there is no necessity to exclude contaminant signals from surrounding tissues[17, 18]. The tissue under study can be positioned in this homogeneous zone, and held rigidly during the study. Finally, a surface coil is positioned so that its sensitive volume encompasses both the required tissue and the homogeneous magnetic volume. All this must be accomplished whilst keeping the patient comfortable and using non-magnetic positioning and supporting mechanisms.

7.3.2. Muscle studies

The bore of the TMR 200/32 magnet (20 cm diameter) restricts muscle examinations mainly to the calf, hand or forearm. In these studies the tissues under investigation lie relatively close to the skin and are separated from the coil by subcutaneous fat and dermal tissues. Muscle is the only ·tissue present containing significant concentrations of phosphorus metabolites and

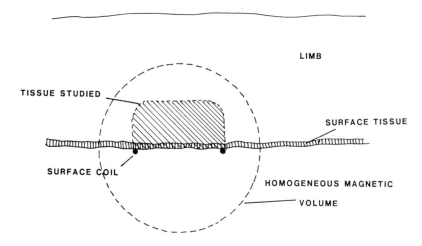

Figure 4. The relative positioning involved in Duchenne dystrophy studies.

it is not essential to use the homogeneous magnetic volume. In studies of Duchenne muscular dystrophy only the shimmed main field is used and the maximum amount of tissue is interrogated by the coil. The relative positioning of coil, limb and homogeneous volume is illustrated schematically in figure 4. Some investigations require the use of the profiling coils in order to eliminate signal from surface tissues (especially in ^{13}C or ^{1}H studies) or to localize the sensitivity to one particular muscle.

In the case of forearm and hand studies, the patient sits alongside the magnet with the outstretched arm in the magnet bore. The arm rests in a padded "U" shaped plastic moulding which has the surface coil mounted in an aperture in the support as illustrated in figure 5. The surface coil is rigidly clamped in the magnet bore so as to achieve the correct positioning with respect to the homogeneous volume. The plastic support can be adjusted vertically and horizontally to accommodate variation in limb size and angle. The arm rest also contains a hand grip with a built in strain gauge force monitor for dynamic exercise studies.

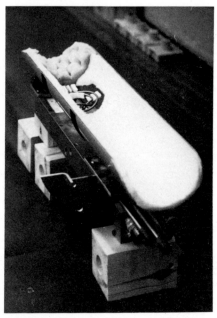

Figure 5. The arm support employed in muscle studies showing the position of the surface coil mounting. The PTFE spacer has been removed for clarity.

In the case of calf muscle, it has been found most convenient to lie patients on their backs on a wooden couch, with the limb under study extended in the magnet bore. The leg is supported in a plastic moulding similar to that used on the arm. In studies of Duchenne muscular dystrophy, the coil is mounted in the same way as for the forearm. In other investigations "flying lead" coils are strapped to the appropriate part of the limb or the coil can be supported on an adjustable frame clamped to the surface of the magnet bore.

In all limb investigations, it is necessary to earth the limb as close as possible to the surface coil. This is achieved using a flexible aluminium foil earthing strap which wraps around the limb using electrode gel as a contact medium and is connected directly to the metal bore of the magnet.

7.3.3. Neonatal brain monitoring

This area of study is the one which presents the greatest technical problems in terms of patient handling. The infants studied are either premature or term and have undergone some degree of asphyxia during or prior to birth. They can be extremely small (< 1 kg) and may require extensive life support measures.

In these cases we have to provide a complete neonatal intensive care system which fits into the bore of the NMR magnet. Such a system must provide firstly, all the monitoring facilities normally encountered in the neonatal intensive care unit, so that the NMRS study will involve no extra risk to the infant. These include ambient temperature control, mechanical ventilation, and monitoring of ECG, breath rate, blood pressure, arterial oxygen tension and skin temperature. The system must, secondly, provide a means of positioning the infant's head and surface coil correctly with respect to the homogeneous magnetic volume. Thirdly, it must provide all these functions while employing no ferromagnetic components inside the magnet and not increasing the RF interference.

The positioning problem in brain studies is complicated by the presence of subcutaneous muscle tissue which would contaminate the results and hence the homogeneous volume must be used. The tissue of interest (brain) is surrounded by a layer of bone and may be a considerable distance from the surface coil. Head diameters vary from 5 to 12 cm and for this reason, we use a surface coil with a diameter (7 cm) greater than that of the homogeneous magnetic volume. The coil is positioned so that the edge of the homogeneous volume is 0.5 cm into the skull. This is designed to exclude signal from the surface tissues and ensure that the resultant spectrum is from brain

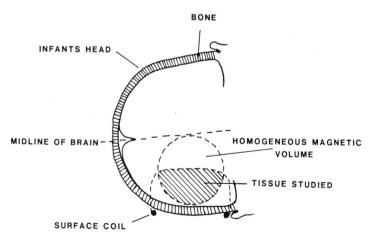

Figure 6. The relative positioning involved in neonatal brain studies.

tissue occupying a large part of the volume interrogated by the coil. The use of a 180° pulse at the surface further reduces possible signal from surface tissues[16]. Figure 6 illustrates the positioning usually employed in these studies.

This positioning is achieved in practice by mounting the surface coil rigidly onto a platform built into a Perspex tube which forms a canopy for the infant. The platform height within the tube is adjustable by means of plastic spacers, and the surface coil is incorporated into a foam pillow on which the infant's head lies. The arrangement is illustrated schematically in figure 7. The Perspex tube, sealed at each end, splits lengthwise so that the

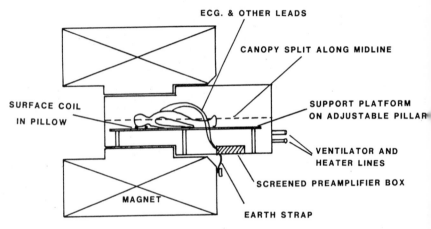

Figure 7. The neonatal canopy in the bore of the magnet.

upper half can be lifted off. Inlets for the ventilator lines and warm air are incorporated in one end. ECG leads and other monitoring instrumentation in the canopy connect to an earthed metallic box and then to a battery operated preamplifier. Here the signals are converted into optical form and transmitted down fibre optics to a decoder placed about three metres away from the magnet alongside the mechanical ventilator and heater. The infant is earthed by a flexible metal braid connected to the screened box containing the preamplifier. This earthing arrangement together with the optical signal coupling has led to the achievement of noise levels near the theoretical minimum.

All the major monitoring and mechanical life support apparatus contains ferromagnetic components and is contained in a standard neonatal transport incubator remote from the magnet. During transport to the magnet, the

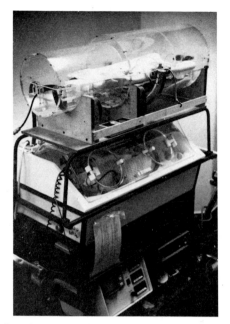

Figure 8. The neonatal canopy mounted for transport on top of a standard neonatal transport incubator.

Perspex canopy clips on top of the incubator. This is shown in figure 8.

7.3.4. *Future developments*

Many problems have still to be solved in the mechanics and monitoring of muscle and brain. In the muscle studies, the problem of noise could be tackled by screening the room containing the magnet, but such a solution would be expensive. The technique of multiple earthing may prove to be an acceptable alternative. Instrumentation for EMG measurement is also required, and will probably have to employ the same optical isolation techniques used for the neonatal monitoring. In the longer term, it would be advantageous in the case of patients with certain pathologies to transport them from the ward to magnet with minimal muscular exertion. This would require the building of a non-magnetic wheelchair so that the patient could be wheeled directly up to the magnet.

For the neonatal brain studies, a non-magnetic transport incubator frame is being built on to which the Perspex canopy will be permanently attached. A revised canopy is also under construction which incorporates all the necessary signal preamplifiers. It is intended that some means of lowering the platform which supports the baby will be incorporated. This would allow different areas of the brain to be studied easily and quickly.

7.4. Clinical results

The main areas of clinical research and routine application of ^{31}P NMRS at University College Hospital (UCH) are muscle disease in children and adults and cerebral metabolism in neonates. The response of a malignant tumour to chemotherapy has been studied; however, tumours are rarely located in a suitable position for investigation in a 20 cm bore magnet.

UCH has many advantages for studies of muscle and cerebral metabolism. The Department of Medicine specializes in metabolic studies of muscle. Clinical back-up is available and there is a particularly strong interest in the muscular dystrophies. Patients are referred from clinics in other parts of the British Isles so that large numbers of investigations have been possible.

The North East Thames Regional Neonatal Unit is at UCH and provides a comprehensive service over a large catchment area providing many cases for study. This allows the correlation of NMRS results with other investigations such as ultrasound. The interpretation of clinical ^{31}P NMRS studies of neonatal cerebral metabolism depends strongly on the availability of routine follow-up for each infant and this service is provided by the Neonatal Unit.

7.4.1. Muscle studies

Before attempting to understand the changes observed in pathological muscle it is necessary to define the characteristics of the normal population. Figures 9(a) and (b) show normal muscle spectra from resting forearm and posterior calf muscles respectively. The most conspicuous feature of the spectra is the large resonance of phosphocreatine (PCr). Downfield from this peak (negative ppm; by convention spectra are presented with the wavelength increasing from left to right) are the three resonances of the γ, α and β phosphorus nuclei of adenosine triphosphate (ATP). (Note the "fine" structure in the ATP resonances caused by spin–spin coupling between the phosphorus nuclei. The γ and α ATP resonances are doublets and the β ATP resonance is a triplet.) ATP and PCr are often termed "high energy" phosphates because they are intimately involved in both cellular energy production and biosynthesis; this is the main reason for focussing attention on them in biochemical studies. The γ ATP peak contains a small contribution from adenosine diphosphate (ADP) and the α ATP contains nicotinamide adenine dinucleotide components (NAD and NADH). Upfield from the PCr, the most conspicuous peak is that of inorganic orthophosphate (Pi) at about $+5$ ppm. Between the Pi and the PCr is the phospho-diester (PD) resonance band. A small PD peak shows up clearly in the calf spectrum (figure 9(b)). Further upfield from the Pi is the sugar phosphate (SP) band. Only a small amount

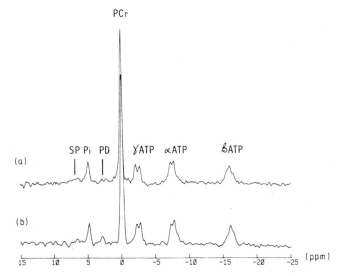

Figure 9. ³¹P NMR spectra of normal, resting, *in vivo* muscle tissue. (a) Forearm muscle, 30 μs pulse, 6 cm surface coil, 512 scans, 2 s pulse delay. (b) Posterior calf muscle (mainly gastrocnemius). 40 μs pulse, 5 cm surface coil (flying lead), 128 scans, 10 s pulse delay (relaxed spectrum).

of SP is found in normal resting muscle. Many metabolites are found to resonate in the PD and SP bands and usually a peak will consist of several, unresolved, overlapping signals.

In order to derive metabolite ratios, the appropriate saturation factors must be applied. These have been determined for muscle tissue examined under our experimental conditions and our reported muscle metabolite levels have been corrected. Concentrations measured relative to a total mobile phosphorus content of 1.00 are shown in table 3. The intracellular pH (defined

Table 3. Comparison of metabolite levels and pH for normal and dystrophic muscle tissue (relative to total phosphorus = 1.00)

	Normal muscle ($n = 24$)		Dystrophic muscle ($n = 55$, 9 individuals)	
	Mean	SD	Mean	SD
pH	7.04	0.05	7.07	0.04
pCr	0.49	0.03	0.39	0.03
Pi	0.08	0.01	0.14	0.02
PD	0.03	0.02	0.07	0.02
ATP	0.11	0.01	0.11	0.01
SP	0.04	0.02	0.06	0.03
NAD + NADH	0.02	0.01	0.02	0.01
PCr/ATP	4.44	0.49	3.72	0.50
PCr/Pi	6.71	1.54	2.89	0.64

as $-\log(H^+)$) can be determined from the chemical shift of the Pi relative to the PCr resonance[4]. The resonant frequencies of many metabolites (excluding PCr) depend on pH and this dependency can be calibrated. For various reasons the Pi peak is the most practicable. Normal adult muscle gives a mean pH of 7.04 (SD = 0.05, $n = 24$). Similarly the ATP resonant frequencies depend on the degree of binding to Mg^{2+} which, in normal muscle, is greater than 90%. The unbound β ATP resonance is about 2 ppm downfield from the bound position[30].

Differences can be anticipated between spectra from different muscles. There are two main types of muscle fibre referred to as types I and II[31, 32]. Type I fibres contain more oxidative enzymes and can sustain a moderate power output without fatigue, whereas type II fibres have high glycolytic enzyme content and can produce a very high power output for "sprint" performance. The distribution of muscle fibre types I and II varies from muscle to muscle and from individual to individual depending appropriately on the function required. This may be reflected in the metabolite concentrations determined by ^{31}P NMRS especially during exercise studies. Biopsy analysis has also shown that the concentration of PD is much greater in the calf than in the forearm[33]. There is also an experimental effect due to anatomical differences that may influence the results. The posterior of the calf contains three large muscle units; the lateral and medial heads of the gastrocnemius, and centrally the soleus muscle. The large sizes of these muscles make it possible to design investigations that obtain spectra from only one particular muscle. This is difficult in the forearm where functional muscle units are small and studies may contain contributions from muscles in both the resting and exercised states.

Much of the muscle research has been devoted to the monitoring of trials in Duchenne muscular dystrophy[34]. This is a severe hereditary muscle disease which affects males at an early age. It has an incidence at birth of about 1/3000 and has a fatal outcome in the second decade of life. The population of Duchenne patients under study at UCH consists of nine boys aged 3 to 13 years. Figures 10(a) and (b) show spectra obtained from the posterior mid-calves of two such patients. There is a significantly large PD peak and the PCr/Pi and PCr/ATP ratios are much smaller than in the normal case. The relative metabolite concentrations are shown in table 3. No significant difference in pH (7.07, SD = 0.04, $n = 55$, nine individuals) has been observed for our population when compared with normals. It has been reported that a difference exists[35] but the spectra shown in the study quoted do not appear to be very well resolved and this can cause shifting of the PCr and Pi peaks. Another reason for discrepancy may be that our patients are young and constitute a sample in which the disease may not be very advanced.

Figures 10(c) and (d) were obtained from a patient with hypothyroid myopathy. Figure 10(c) was obtained before beginning a course of L-thyroxine therapy and exhibits a strong resonance in the PD band (about 3 ppm) which appears to be characteristic of this disease[6]. Figure 10(d) shows a previously

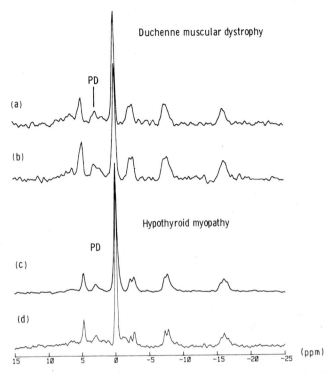

Figure 10. ³¹P NMR spectra of pathological, resting, *in vivo* muscle tissue. (a) and (b). Spectra from the posterior calf muscles of two individuals with Duchenne muscular dystrophy. Note the presence of a strong PD signal and the lower PCr/Pi and PCr/ATP ratios. 30 μs pulse, 6 cm surface coil, 512 scans, 2 s pulse delay. (c) Forearm spectrum from a case of hypothyroid myopathy before treatment. Note the presence of a PD resonance. 30 μs pulse, 6 cm surface coil, 320 scans, 2 s pulse delay. (d) Similar to (c) but one day after commencement of L-thyroxine therapy and 768 scans. PD resonance is still detected and an unknown resonance appears at about −1 ppm.

undetected resonance at about −1 ppm a few days after starting treatment.

Many metabolic defects that ³¹P NMRS is capable of investigating are only revealed when muscle is exercised and metabolic pathways are tested. One routine way of doing this is to demand a maximal amount of effort from the muscle and then to trap the metabolites by applying an ischaemic cuff. The effort usually consists of a 60 s maximal voluntary isometric contraction and before termination of this the cuff is applied in a rapid but controlled way using compressed air, thereby avoiding nervous damage and stopping venous and arterial flow simultaneously. Monitoring of the metabolite levels is achieved by sequential data acquisitions (see figures 11(a) to

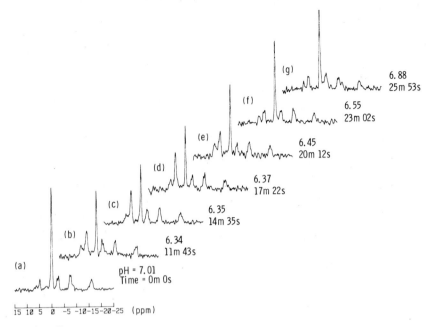

Figure 11. ^{31}P NMR spectra of normal *in vivo* muscle tissue undergoing exercise. (a) Resting spectrum. (b), (c) and (d). Spectra with ischaemic cuff applied after a 60 s maximal voluntary contraction (MVC). (e) (f) and (g). Recovery sequence with ischaemic cuff off. Times of data acquisition and measured pH are shown. 30 µs pulse, 6 cm surface coil, 64 scans, 2 s pulse delay.

(g)) which are of one or two minutes duration starting with resting spectra as a baseline for comparison. Usually two or three spectra are collected during ischaemia and then the cuff is released and several spectra are obtained until the muscle has recovered its normal, resting state. During exercise the Pi increases rapidly and the increase is maintained when the cuff is applied. This is accompanied by a marked decrease in the PCr and a slight increase in the SP. Accompanying these changes is an acid shift (downfield) of the Pi resonance caused by the production of lactic acid as a result of glycolysis (the metabolic pathway by which glycogen is broken down to produce ATP). The normal resting pH is about 7.0 but after exercise this may fall to as low as 6.3. Certain enzyme defects can reveal themselves in exercise studies. McArdle's syndrome manifests itself as an inability to produce lactic acid so no fall in pH is observed after exercise. In fact a slight alkaline shift is seen as a result of the hydrolysis of PCr to creatine (Cr) and Pi which is a process that consumes H^+[36]. Phosphofructokinase (PFK) deficiency leads to the production of large amounts of hexose monophosphate during exercise which cannot be further converted to fructose 1:6 diphosphate because the appropriate enzyme (PFK) is virtually absent. The build up of hexose monophosphate is revealed by the presence of a large SP peak during exercise. Many different pathologies have been investigated using this technique, including hypothyroid myopathy and muscular dystrophy.

Examples of spectra from neonatal muscle are shown in figures 12(a)

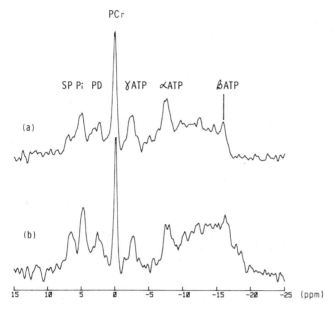

Figure 12. (a) and (b) ^{31}P NMR spectra of neonatal muscle (mainly gluteus maximus) from two infants. 15 μs pulse, 3 cm surface coil, 512 scans, 2 s pulse delay. Note the high SP, Pi and PD levels and the conspicuous, broad signal between the α and β ATP resonances (probably due to phospholipids).

and (b). These were obtained from infants with cerebral lesions and presumably represent normal muscle. Considerable differences are apparent when these spectra are compared with the normal adult muscles shown in figure 9(a) and (b).

7.4.2. Studies of neonatal cerebral metabolism

The pathologies studied have, in general, been those that compromise, acutely or chronically, the oxygenation of the brain tissue. Similar to the effect of ischaemia on muscle, this has a profound effect on certain of the phosphorus metabolites, particularly the PCr and Pi[37] and possibly on the pH[38]. Pathologies investigated have included birth asphyxia, postnatal asphyxial episodes, intraventricular haemorrhage (IVH), metabolic defects, meningitis and hydrocephalus. Many cases are referred when routine ultrasound scans show signs of IVH, enlarged ventricles or development of cysts. About 30 infants have been studied and some have been investigated on more than one occasion enabling the monitoring of recovery and the evaluation of various regimes of therapy. Many lesions are global, in which case usually only one cerebral hemisphere is studied. Sometimes ultrasound or other examination indicates an asymmetric pathology and both hemispheres are examined[37]. Saturation factors for most of the brain spectra discussed are not yet available and reported metabolite levels may need reviewing in the near future.

Figure 13(a) is an example of a fully relaxed spectrum (pulse delay 20 s)

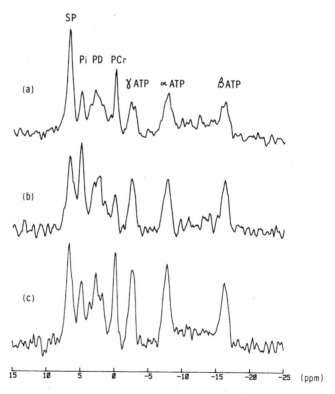

Figure 13. ^{31}P NMR spectra of neonatal *in vivo* brain tissue. (a) A fully relaxed spectrum of normal brain. 100 μs pulse, 7 cm surface coil, 128 scans, 20 s pulse delay. (b) and (c) Spectra from an infant that suffered a severe asphyxial episode after birth. Spectrum (b) was obtained shortly after the insult and (c) approximately two weeks later. Acquisition parameters similar to (a) but 1024 scans, 2 s pulse delay. Note the recovery of the PCr and the drop in Pi level in spectrum (c).

obtained from a normal infant. ATP, PCr and Pi are present but in different relative amounts compared with normal muscle. A large signal is seen in the PD region which probably originates from several, unresolved, overlapping resonances. The most prominent feature is in the SP band and has been tentatively identified as a ribose-5-phosphate[37, 39]. For this spectrum, the metabolite ratios (relative to total phosphorus = 1.00) are SP = 0.24, Pi = 0.08, PD = 0.22, PCr = 0.11 and ATP = 0.12. The ratios PCr/Pi and PCR/ATP are considered to be indicators of the metabolic state and in this case are 1.32 and 0.89 respectively. The pH determined from the PCr and Pi chemical shift is 7.2. Some reports of mammalian brain spectra show larger amounts of PCr and less SP than we have found[39-42]. This may be due to contamination of the signal with subcutaneous muscle (high PCr, low SP), to the fact that previous studies have looked at "whole" brain, whereas for experimental reasons we may have studied mainly the cerebral cortex (grey matter), or the high SP may be a feature of neonatal metabolism. By judicious selection of pulse length[16] and coil position relative to the homogeneous volume, contamination of our results by muscle signal has been minimized. Figure 13(b) is a spectrum from an infant who suffered a severe asphyxial episode a few days after birth. The spectrum was obtained at age two days and is remarkable for the large Pi and low PCr levels, which are indicative of this kind of lesion. A spectrum at age 15 days is shown in figure 13(c) and the PCr has recovered at the expense of the Pi. The inference from this is that remaining viable brain tissue is recovering from the asphyxial insult. During the interval between examinations the PCr/ATP changed from 0.44 to 0.82, the PCr/Pi from 0.37 to 1.26 and the pH dropped from 7.4 to 7.0.

Two infants with metabolic defects (propionic acidaemia and arginosuccinic aciduria) have been studied (figures 14(a), (b) and (c), (d) respectively). Striking differences are apparent between these and the normal spectrum shown in figure 13(a). The PCr and ATP are almost completely undetectable whereas the Pi resonance now dominates the spectrum. Upfield from the Pi a SP resonance is situated at about 7 ppm and a PD peak is present near 2.5 ppm. The spectra strongly resemble those obtained previously from hypoxic mammalian brain tissue[40-43]. Both infants died shortly after examination. The pH of the tissue was determined by use of the H_2O resonance as a reference[14] and a strong acid Pi shift was found (pH = 6.5, SD = 0.1, $n = 4$). The use of the H_2O resonance as a reference for pH determination in ^{31}P brain spectra has been very useful in cases of low or absent PCr signal. Results obtained and tests on other tissues with strong PCr signals indicate that in cases of high PCr the technique is as good as using the PCr as a reference. For low PCr the method is much better and sometimes (see figure 14) is the only method by which pH can be determined.

Figures 15(a) to (e) show a sequence of spectra taken in a case of birth asphyxia from age 42 hours (a) to age 26 days (e). The sequence shows initially high Pi and low PCr levels which, by day 26, are more normal. Ultrasound

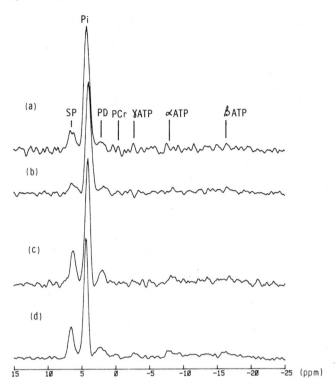

Figure 14. ^{31}P NMR brain spectra of two infants with metabolic defects. (a) and (b) are from a neonate with propionic acidaemia and were obtained from the same hemisphere on two consecutive days. Acquisition parameters as for figures 5(b) and (c) but with 512 scans. (c) and (d) are from a case of arginosuccinic aciduria. They were acquired on the same day from the left and right hemispheres respectively. Acquisition parameters as for figure 5(b) and (c) but spectrum (c) has 512 scans. Note the almost undetectable PCr and ATP levels in all these spectra.

examination showed the development of porencephalic cysts at age 20 days. The pH was slightly alkaline throughout the series.

7.4.3. Monitoring of tumour chemotherapy

An opportunity to study a malignant tumour occurred when a patient was referred to UCH with a rhabdomyosarcoma on the dorsum of the hand[44]. Figures 16(b) and (c) show spectra obtained on two separate occasions before and after a course of chemotherapy. Figure 16(a) shows a spectrum from the dorsum of a normal hand for comparison. The tumour spectra are very different from the normal spectrum, which arises mainly from the inter-osseous

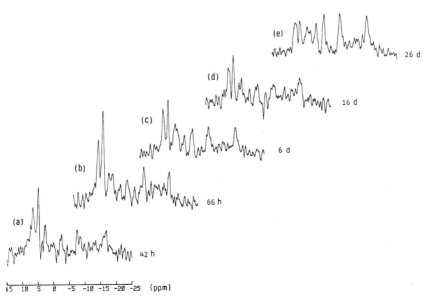

Figure 15. A sequence of ³¹P NMR spectra from a birth asphyxiated infant. The spectra were obtained at intervals from age 42 hours to 26 days and acquisition parameters were similar to those for figures 5(b) and (c).

muscles and they show a strong resemblance to the brain spectra described previously. Figure 16(c) was obtained two months after figure 16(b), during which time the patient's condition had deteriorated and a third examination was impossible. The main difference between the two tumour spectra is a fall in the PCr seen in the second spectrum. Measurement of the integral showed that PCr/ATP had fallen to 75% and PCr/Pi to 70% of their previous values. It has been reported that PCr levels fall as tumour development occurs because the cells become anoxic[45]. The intracellular pH was found to be 7.1 and very similar to that found in animal tumours[6]. The rarity of suitable patients has meant that no opportunity has arisen for determining saturation factors for metabolites in tumour tissue.

The effectiveness of the various anticarcinogenic drugs is hard to assess using unaided clinical criteria. ³¹P NMRS provides the possibility that we may arrive, more quickly than at present, at the method of treatment that best suits the needs of each individual patient. The critical outcome for the patient of successfully applied therapy is so important that ³¹P NMRS must be considered as a potential monitoring method especially when "whole body" systems become readily available.

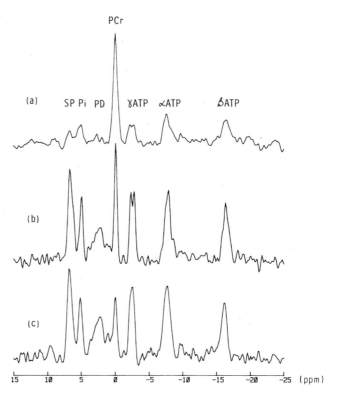

Figure 16. ^{31}P NMR spectra of normal hand and rhabdomyosarcoma *in situ*. (a) Normal hand spectrum which consists mainly of signal from inter-osseous muscle. 24 μs pulse, 4 cm surface coil, 128 scans, 2 s pulse delay. (b) Rhabdomyosarcoma spectrum obtained before commencing a course of chemotherapy. (c) Spectrum from same tumour acquired two months later. Acquisition parameters for (b) and (c) are the same as for (a) but 512 scans. A marked decrease in the PCr level is seen in spectrum (c).

References

1. Gordon R E 1981 From molecules to man: NMR finds a new application *Physics Bulletin* **32** 178–180
2. National Radiological Protection Board 1980 Exposure to nuclear magnetic resonance clinical imaging *Radiography* **47** 258–261
3. Food and Drug Administration USA 1982 *Guidelines for evaluating electromagnetic exposure risk for trials of clinical NMR systems* (Washington: Public Health Services)
4. Moon R B and Richards J H 1973 Determination of intracellular pH by ^{31}P magnetic resonance *Journal of Biological Chemistry* **248** 7276–7278
5. O'Neill I K and Richards C P 1980 Biological ^{31}P NMR spectroscopy *Annual Reports on NMR Spectroscopy* **10A** 133–247

6. Iles R A, Stevens A N and Griffiths J R 1982 NMR studies of metabolites in living tissue *Progress in NMR Spectroscopy* **15** 49–200
7. Alger J R, Sillerud L O, Behar K L, Gillies R J, Shulman R G, Gordon R E, Shaw D and Hanley P E 1981 *In vivo* carbon-13 nuclear magnetic resonance studies of mammals *Science* **214** 660–662
8. Ackermann J J H, Grove T H, Wong G G, Gadian D G and Radda G K 1980 Mapping of metabolites in whole animals by ^{31}P NMR using surface coils *Nature* **283** 167–170
9. Griffiths J R and Iles R A 1980 Nuclear magnetic resonance—a 'magnetic eye' on metabolism *Clinical Science* **59** 225–230
10. Gadian D G 1982 *Nuclear Magnetic Resonance and its Application to Living Systems* (Oxford: Clarendon Press)
11. Abragam A 1961 *The Principles of Nuclear Magnetism* (Oxford: Clarendon Press)
12. Slichter C P 1978 *Principles of Magnetic Resonance*, 2nd edn (Berlin: Springer Verlag)
13. Becker E D 1980 *High Resolution NMR* (New York: Academic Press)
14. Ackerman J J H, Gadian D G, Radda G K and Wong G G 1980 Observation of ^1H NMR signals with receiver coils tuned for other nuclides *Journal of Magnetic Resonance* **42** 498–500
15. Gordon R E and Timms W E 1982 An improved tune and match circuit for B_0 shimming in intact biological samples. *Journal of Magnetic Resonance* **46** 322–324
16. Balaban R S, Gadian D G and Radda G K 1981 Phosphorus nuclear magnetic resonance study of the rat kidney in vivo *Kidney International* **20** 575–579
17. Gordon R E, Hanley P E, Shaw D, Gadian D G, Radda G K, Styles P, Bore P J and Chan L 1980 Localisation of metabolites in animals using ^{31}P topical magnetic resonance *Nature* **287** 736–738
18. Gordon R E, Hanley P E and Shaw D 1982 Topical magnetic resonance *Progress in NMR Spectroscopy* **15** 1–47
19. Becker E D, Ferretti J A and Gambhir P N 1979 Selection of optimum parameters for pulse fourier transform nuclear magnetic resonance *Analytical Chemistry* **51** 1413–1420
20. Waugh J S 1970 Sensitivity in fourier transform NMR spectroscopy of slowly relaxing systems *Journal of Molecular Spectroscopy* **35** 298–305
21. Ernst R R and Anderson W A 1966 Application of Fourier transform spectroscopy to magnetic resonance *Review of Scientific Instruments* **37** 93–102
22. Hoult D I 1978 The NMR receiver: A description and analysis of design *Progress in NMR Spectroscopy* **12** 41–77
23. Lindon J C and Ferrige A G 1980 Digitisation and data processing in Fourier transform NMR *Progress in NMR Spectroscopy* **14** 27–66
24. Hoult D I and Richards R E 1976 The signal to noise ratio of the Nuclear Magnetic Resonance Experiment *Journal of Magnetic Resonance* **24** 71–85
25. Gadian D G and Robinson F N H 1979 Radiofrequency losses in NMR experiments on electrically conducting samples *Journal of Magnetic Resonance* **34** 449–455
26. Bleaney B I and Bleaney B 1965 *Electricity and Magnetism* (Oxford University Press) p. 150
27. Smythe W R 1950 *Static and Dynamic Electricity* (New York: McGraw Hill) p. 318
28. Mansfield P and Morris P G 1982 NMR Imaging in Biomedicine. In *Advances in Magnetic Resonance* (New York: Academic Press) p. 294
29. Bottomley P A and Andrew E R 1978 RF magnetic field penetration, phase shift and power dissipation in biological tissue: Implications for NMR imaging *Physics in Medicine and Biology* **23** 630–643
30. Cohn M and Hughes T R 1962 Nuclear magnetic resonance spectra of adenosine di- and triphosphate *Journal of Biological Chemistry* **237** 176–181
31. Buchthal F and Schmalbruch H 1970 Contraction times and fibre types in intact human muscle *Acta Physiologica Scandinavica* **79** 435–452
32. Essen B, Janssen E, Henriksson J, Taylor A W and Saltin B 1975 Metabolic characteristics of fibre types in human skeletal muscle *Acta Physiologica Scandinavica* **95** 153–165

33. Edwards R H T, Dawson M J, Wilkie D R, Gordon R E and Shaw D 1982 Clinical use of nuclear magnetic resonance in the investigation of myopathy *Lancet* **1** 725
34. Gardner-Medwin D 1980 Clinical features and classification of muscular dystrophies *British Medical Bulletin* **36**(2) 109–115
35. Newman R J, Bore P J, Chan L, Gadian D G, Styles P, Taylor D and Radda G K 1982 Nuclear magnetic resonance studies of forearm muscle in Duchenne dystrophy *British Medical Journal* **284** 1072–1074
36. Radda G K, Gadian D G and Ross B D 1982 Energy metabolism and cellular pH in normal and pathological conditions. A new look through 31 phosphorus nuclear magnetic resonance. In *Metabolic Acidosis* (London: Pitman) CIBA Foundation symposium 87, p. 36–57
37. Cady E B, Costellow A M de L, Dawson M J, Delpy D T, Hope P L, Reynolds E O R, Tofts P S and Wilkie D R 1983 Non-invasive investigation of cerebral metabolism in newborn infants by phosphorus nuclear magnetic resonance spectroscopy *Lancet* **1** 1059
38. Petroff O A C and Prichard J W 1983 Cerebral pH by NMR *Lancet* **2** 105–106
39. Glonek T, Kopp S J, Kot E, Pettegrew J W, Harrison W H and Cohen M M 1982 ^{31}P nuclear magnetic resonance analysis of brain: the perchloric acid extract spectrum *Journal of Neurochemistry* **39** 1210–1219
40. Delpy D T, Gordon R E, Hope P L, Parker D, Reynolds E O R, Shaw D and Whitehead M D 1982 Non-invasive investigation of cerebral ischaemia by phosphorus nuclear magnetic resonance *Pediatrics* **70** 310–313
41. Thulborn K R, du Boulay G H, Duchen L W and Radda G K 1982 A ^{31}P nuclear magnetic resonance in vivo study of cerebral ischaemia in the gerbil *Journal of Cerebral Blood Flow Metabolism* **2** 299–306
42. Chance B, Nakase Y, Bond M, Leigh J S and McDonald G 1978 Detection of ^{31}P nuclear magnetic resonance signals in brain by in vivo and freeze trapped assays. *Proceedings of the National Academy of Science, USA* **75** 4925–4929
43. Cox D W G, Morris P G, Feeney J and Bachelard H S 1983 ^{31}P NMR studies on cerebral energy metabolism under conditions of hypoglycaemia and hypoxia in vitro *Biochemical Journal* **212** 365–370
44. Griffiths J R, Cady E, Edwards R H T, McCready V R, Wilkie D R and Wiltshaw E 1983 ^{31}P NMR studies of a human tumour in situ *Lancet* **1** 1435–1436
45. Ng T C, Evanochko W T, Hiramoto R N, Ghanta V K, Lilly M B, Lawson A J, Corbett T H, Durant J R and Glickson J D 1982 ^{31}P NMR spectroscopy of in vivo tumours *Journal of Magnetic Resonance* **49** 271–286

CHAPTER **8 Introductory bibliography**

K Straughan

Department of Medical Physics, Hammersmith Hospital,
Du Cane Rd,
London W12 0HS, England

8.1. Introduction

The literature on NMR imaging and related topics has reached large propor-
tions, thus presenting a rather daunting prospect to interested researchers.
Because no book of this size could attempt to give more than an introduction
to this new modality and some of its applications, it was anticipated that
the inclusion of a bibliography would assist the reader. The result, presented
here, is not comprehensive but it is hoped that the references cited will provide
a useful framework for study.

The references concentrate almost entirely on the physical and technical
aspects of the subject. Those subject areas which are covered in the main
body of this book contain their own references.

To facilitate use, the references have been split into a number of sections,
each containing references which range from introductory works to recent,
more advanced research papers, in that order. An additional section contains
a selection of textbooks relating to the theory of NMR and its biological
and clinical applications.

The highly multidisciplinary nature of clinical NMR is reflected in the
wide range of journals from which the citations have been drawn. A list of
these journals is presented below.

Advances in Magnetic Resonance
American Journal of Roentgenology
Annali dell' Istituto Superiore di Sanità
Annals of the New York Academy of Sciences
Biochimica et Biophysica Acta
Biochemical Society Transactions
British Journal of Cancer
British Journal of Radiology
Cancer
Computers in Biology and Medicine
CT: the Journal of Computed Tomography
Current Topics in Membranes and Transport
Electromedica
Frontiers of Biological Energetics
IEEE Transactions on Biomedical
  Engineering

IEEE Transactions on Medical Imaging
IEEE Transactions on Nuclear Science
Journal of Applied Physics
Journal of Computer Assisted Tomography
Journal of Magnetic Resonance
Journal of Nuclear Medicine
Journal of Physical Chemistry
Journal of Physics C: Solid State Physics
Journal of Physics E: Scientific Instruments
Journal of the Physical Society of Japan
Journal of Pure and Applied Chemistry
Journal of Scientific Instruments
Magnetic Resonance Imaging
Medical Physics
Molecular Physics
Nature

Noninvasive Medical Imaging
Nuovo Cimento
Physics in Medicine and Biology
Physics Letters
Physical Review
Physiological Chemistry and Physics
Proceedings of the Indian Academy of
 Science
Proceedings of the National Academy of
 Science of the USA
Proceedings of the Royal Society of London:
 Series B

Proceedings of the Society of Photo-Optical
 Instrumentation Engineers: Application of
 Optical Instrumentation in Medicine IX
Progress in Biophysics and Molecular
 Biology
Progress in Nuclear Magnetic Resonance
 Spectroscopy
Radiography
Radiology
Review of Scientific Instruments
Science

8.2. General NMR texts

To date, there are very few texts devoted entirely to NMR imaging, and those that are available are, in the main, multi-author conglomerates. Also, because of the extremely rapid development of the subject, the books do not contain state-of-the-art information. Nevertheless, they do serve as valuable introductory material. The book by Mansfield and Morris is the only one currently available which gives a physical and mathematical treatment of the subject in any great depth.

In contrast, NMR in general is extremely well served by textbooks, although most of them are heavily biased towards spectroscopic NMR and, as such, are of limited interested to the reader interested in imaging. Several texts are listed below, however, which might be of use in understanding the theory and some biological applications of NMR.

Partain C L, James A E, Rollo F D and Price R R (eds) 1983 *Nuclear Magnetic Resonance (NMR) Imaging* (Philadelphia: Saunders)
Kaufman L, Margulis A R and Crooks L E (eds) 1981 *Nuclear Magnetic Resonance Imaging in Medicine* (New York: Igaku-Schoin)
Mansfield P and Morris P G 1983 *NMR Imaging in Biomedicine. Supplement 2. Advances in Magnetic Resonance* (New York: Academic Press)
Gadian D G 1982 *Nuclear Magnetic Resonance and its Applications to Living Systems* (Oxford: Clarendon Press)
Fukushima E and Roeder S B W 1981 *Experimental Pulse NMR. A Nuts and Bolts Approach* (New York: Addison-Wesley)
Farrar T C and Becker E D 1971 *Pulse and Fourier Transform NMR (Introduction to Theory and Methods)* (New York: Academic Press)
Slichter C P 1963 *Principles of Magnetic Resonance* (New York: Harper and Row) (2nd edition, 1978, Springer-Verlag, Berlin)
Shaw D 1976 *Fourier Transform NMR Spectroscopy* (Amsterdam: Elsevier/North Holland)
Andrew E R 1969 *Nuclear Magnetic Resonance* (Cambridge University Press)
Abragam A 1961 *The Principles of Nuclear Magnetism* (Oxford: Clarendon Press)

8.3. NMR theory

We present here only a few of the many relevant publications, chosen to cover the major historical discoveries which are now utilized in NMR imaging. For those wishing to read further, the book by Abragam (previous section) should provide a good pointer for further study.

Dixon R L and Ekstrand K E 1982 The physics of proton NMR *Medical Physics* **9** 807–818
Bloch F 1946 Nuclear induction *Physical Review* **70** 460–474
Bloch F, Hansen W W and Packard M 1946 The nuclear induction experiment *Physical Review* **70** 474–485
Purcell E M, Torrey H C and Pound R V 1946 Resonance absorption by nuclear magnetic moments in a solid *Physical Review* **69** 37–38
Bloembergen N, Purcell E M and Pound R V 1948 Relaxation effects in nuclear magnetic resonance absorption *Physical Review* **73** 679–712
Hahn E L 1950 Spin–echoes *Physical Review* **80** 580–594
Carr H Y 1958 Steady-state free precession in nuclear magnetic resonance *Physical Review* **112** 1693–1701
Ernst R R and Anderson W A 1966 Application of Fourier Transform spectroscopy to magnetic resonance *Review of Scientific Instruments* **37** 93–102
Jones D E and Sternlicht N 1972 Fourier Transform NMR. 1. Repetitive pulses *Journal of Magnetic Resonance* **6** 167–182
Soda G and Chihara H 1974 Note on the theory of nuclear spin relaxation. Exact formulae in the weak collision limit *Journal of the Physical Society of Japan* **36** 954–958

8.4. NMR imaging: principles and methods

One of the many attractions of NMR imaging, from both a practical and an intellectual viewpoint, is the diversity of imaging regimes which can be implemented. Each regime brings with it its own peculiarities, its own technological requirements, and its own set of advantages and disadvantages. To the uninitiated, as well as to the experienced worker, this can present a nightmare of problems in trying to understand the physics of NMR imaging. This section, and the next, are designed to help.

In this section, a selection of basic introductory works is presented, each giving rather different but lucid explanations of the "nuts and bolts" of the imaging modality. These are followed by some historical papers which follow the development of NMR imaging from its conception in 1973 to the early 1980s and which reveal how the various different techniques have evolved one from another. The section concludes with papers describing progress in recent years up to the current state-of-the-art, together with a selection of advanced papers discussing the physics of the various imaging regimes in greater depth.

References to the theory of image reconstruction for each of the regimes are left, in the main, to section 8.5. Technical and engineering aspects of the implementation of NMR imaging systems are referenced in section 8.6.

Pykett I L, Newhouse J H, Buonanno F S, Brady T J, Goldman M R, Kistler J P and Pohost G M 1982 Principles of nuclear magnetic resonance imaging *Radiology* **143** 157–168
Fullerton G D 1982 Basic concepts for nuclear magnetic resonance imaging *Magnetic Resonance Imaging* **1** 39–55

Lerski R A 1983 Physical principles of nuclear magnetic resonance imaging *Radiography* **49** 85–90

Lauterbur P C 1973 Image formation by induced local interactions: examples employing nuclear magnetic resonance *Nature* **242** 190–191

Lauterbur P C 1974 Magnetic resonance zeugmatography *Journal of Pure and Applied Chemistry* **40** 149–157

Hinshaw W S 1974 Spin mapping: the application of moving gradients to NMR *Physics Letters* **48A** 87–88

Garroway A N, Grannell P K and Mansfield P 1974 Image formation in NMR by a selective irradiation process *Journal of Physics C: Solid State Physics* **7** L457–L462

Grannell P K and Mansfield P 1975 Microscopy in vivo by nuclear magnetic resonance *Physics in Medicine and Biology* **20** 477–482

Mansfield P and Grannell P K 1975 "Diffraction" and microscopy in solids and liquids by NMR *Physical Review* B **12** 3618–3634

Kumar A, Welti D and Ernst R R 1975 NMR Fourier zeugmatography *Journal of Magnetic Resonance* **18** 69–83

Damadian R, Minkoff L, Goldsmith M, Stanford M and Koutcher J 1976 Field focusing nuclear magnetic resonance (FONAR): Visualisation of a tumour in a live animal *Science* **194** 1430–1431

Damadian R, Minkoff L, Goldsmith M, Stanford M and Koutcher J 1976 Tumour imaging in a live animal of Field Focusing NMR (FONAR) *Physiological Chemistry and Physics* **8** 61–65

Mansfield P and Maudsley A A 1976 Planar spin imaging by NMR *Journal of Physics C: Solid State Physics* **9** L409–L412

Hinshaw W S 1976 Image formation by nuclear magnetic resonance: the sensitive point method *Journal of Applied Physics* **47** 3709–3721

Mansfield P and Maudsley A A 1976 Line scan proton spin imaging in biological structures by NMR *Physics in Medicine and Biology* **21** 847–852

Holland G N, Bottomley P A and Hinshaw W S 1977 ^{19}F magnetic resonance imaging *Journal of Magnetic Resonance* **28** 113–136

Mansfield P 1977 Multi-planar image formation using NMR spin echoes *Journal of Physics C: Solid State Physics* **10** L55–L58

Hinshaw W S, Bottomley P A and Holland G N 1977 Radiographic thin-section image of the human wrist by nuclear magnetic resonance *Nature* **270** 722–723

Mansfield P and Maudsley A A 1977 Medical imaging by NMR *British Journal of Radiology* **50** 188–194

Mansfield P and Maudsley A A 1977 Planar spin imaging by NMR *Journal of Magnetic Resonance* **27** 101–119

Hutchison J M S, Sutherland R J and Mallard J R 1978 NMR imaging: image recovery under magnetic fields with large non-uniformities *Journal of Physics E: Scientific Instruments* **11** 217–221

Sutherland R J and Hutchison J M S 1978 Three-dimensional NMR imaging using selective excitation *Journal of Physics E: Scientific Instruments* **11** 79–83

Mansfield P and Pykett I L 1978 Biological and medical imaging by NMR *Journal of Magnetic Resonance* **29** 355–373

Mallard J, Hutchison J M S, Edelstein W A, Ling C R, Foster M A and Johnson G 1980 In vivo n.m.r. imaging in medicine: the Aberdeen approach, both physical and biological *Philosophical Transactions of the Royal Society of London*, Series B **289** S19–S33

Edelstein W A, Hutchison J M S, Johnson G and Redpath T 1980 Spin warp NMR imaging and applications to human whole-body imaging *Physics in Medicine and Biology* **25** 751–756

Ordidge R J, Mansfield P, Doyle M and Coupland R E 1982 Real time movie images by NMR *British Journal of Radiology* **55** 729–733

Maudsley A A 1980 Multiple-line-scanning spin density imaging *Journal of Magnetic Resonance* **41** 112–126

Moore W S and Holland G N 1980 Experimental considerations in implementing a whole body multiple sensitive point nuclear magnetic resonance imaging system *Philosophical Transactions of the Royal Society of London, Series B* **289** 511–518

Bottomley P A 1979 A comparative evaluation of proton NMR imaging results *Journal of Magnetic Resonance* **36** 121–127

Holland G N, Moore W S and Hawkes R C 1981 Nuclear magnetic resonance (NMR) tomography at Nottingham: methods, system technology and results *Proceedings of the Society of Photo-Optical Instrumentation Engineers: Application of Optical Instrumentation in Medicine IX* **273** 2–7

Crooks L E, Herfkens R and Davis P L 1981 Nuclear magnetic resonance (NMR) imaging at the University of California, San Francisco *Proceedings of the Society of Photo-Optical Instrumentation Engineers: Application of Optical Instrumentation in Medicine IX* **273** 11–15

Gore J C, Doyle F H and Pennock J M 1981 Nuclear magnetic resonance (NMR) imaging at Hammersmith Hospital *Proceedings of the Society of Photo-Optical Instrumentation Engineers: Application of Optical Instrumentation in Medicine IX* **273** 8–10

Simon H E 1981 A whole body nuclear magnetic resonance (NMR) imaging system with full three-dimensional capabilities *Proceedings of the Society of Photo-Optical Instrumentation Engineers: Application of Optical Instrumentation in Medicine IX* **273** 41–49

Crooks L, Arakawa M, Hoenninger J, Watts J, McRee R, Kaufman L, Davis P L, Margulis A R and DeGroot J 1982 Nuclear magnetic resonance whole-body imager operating at 3.5 kGauss *Radiology* **143** 169–174

Hoult D I 1979 Rotating frame zeugmatography *Journal of Magnetic Resonance* **33** 183–197

Mansfield P 1981 Critical evaluation of NMR imaging techniques *Proceedings of an International Symposium on Nuclear Magnetic Resonance Imaging, Winston-Salem, North Carolina, USA* (Bowman Gray School of Medicine Press) pp. 81–87

Crooks L E, Mills C M, Davis P L, Brant-Zawadzki M, Hoenninger J, Arakawa M, Watts J and Kaufman L 1982 Visualisation of cerebral and vascular abnormalities by NMR imaging. The effects of imaging parameters on contrast. *Radiology* **144** 843–852

Wehrli F W. MacFall J R and Newton T H 1983 Parameters Determining the Appearance of NMR Images. *Advanced Imaging Techniques, vol. 2* (Modern Neuroradiology series), eds. Newton and Potts (San Anselmo, CA: Clavadel Press) pp. 81–117

Libove J M and Singer J R 1980 Resolution and signal-to-noise relationships in NMR imaging in the human body *Journal of Physics E: Scientific Instruments* **13** 38–44

Brunner P and Ernst R R 1979 Sensitivity and performance time in NMR imaging *Journal of Magnetic Resonance* **33** 83–106

Hoult D I and Lauterbur P C 1979 The sensitivity of the zeugmatographic experiment involving human samples *Journal of Magnetic Resonance* **34** 425–433

Hoult D I 1977 Zeugmatography: a criticism of the concept of a selective pulse in the presence of a field gradient *Journal of Magnetic Resonance* **26** 165–167

Mansfield P, Maudsley A A, Morris P G and Pykett I L 1979 Selective pulses in NMR imaging: a reply to criticism *Journal of Magnetic Resonance* **33** 261–274

Hoult D I 1979 The solution of the Bloch equation in the presence of a varying B_1 field— an approach to selective pulse analysis *Journal of Magnetic Resonance* **35** 67–83

Locher P R 1980 Computer simulation of selective excitation in n.m.r. imaging *Philosophical Transactions of the Royal Society of London Series B* **289** 537–542

Louis A K 1982 Optimal sampling in nuclear magnetic resonance imaging *Journal of Computer Assisted Tomography* **6** 334–340

Johnson G, Hutchison J M S, Redpath T W and Eastwood L M 1983 Improvements in performance time for simultaneous three-dimensional NMR imaging *Journal of Magnetic Resonance* **54** 374–384

Twieg D B 1983 The k-trajectory formulation of the NMR imaging process with applications in analysis and synthesis of imaging methods *Medical Physics* **10** 610–621

Tan H 1981 Nuclear spin density wave mapping by NMR time-axis zeugmatography *Journal of Magnetic Resonance* **45** 356–358

Brown T R, Kincaid B M and Ugurbil K 1982 NMR chemical shift imaging in three dimensions in vivo biochemistry/^{31}P imaging/metabolite mapping) *Proceedings of the National Academy of Sciences of the USA* **79** 3523–3526

Parker D L, Smith V, Sheldon P, Crooks L E and Fussell L 1983 Temperature distribution measurements in two-dimensional NMR imaging *Medical Physics* **10** 321–325

Schneiders N J 1983 Accurate T_2 NMR images *Medical Physics* **10** 642–645

Macovski A 1982 Selective projection imaging: applications to radiography and NMR *IEEE Transactions on Medical Imaging* **MI–1** 42–47

James A E, Partain C L, Holland G N, Gore J C, Rollo F D, Harms S E and Price R R 1981 Nuclear magnetic resonance imaging: the current state *American Journal of Roentgenology* **138** 201–210

Loeffler W and Oppelt A 1982 Possibilities and limitations on NMR imaging *Electromedica* **2/82** 38–40

Crooks L, Arakawa M, Hoenninger J, McCarten B, Watts J and Kaufman L 1984 Magnetic resonance imaging: effects of magnetic field strength *Radiology* **151** 127–133

Axel L 1984 Surface coil magnetic resonance imaging *Journal of Computer Assisted Tomography* **8** 381–384

8.5. Image reconstruction theory

The most commonly known (and understood) reconstruction technique to the medical imaging audience is the projection-reconstruction method. Many of the early commercial NMR scanners utilized this technique, and therefore this section begins with references describing the basics of projection reconstruction. However, the Fourier reconstruction techniques are, in many respects, more attractive for NMR imaging than is projection-reconstruction, so this section goes on to present papers which describe the fundamentals of Fourier reconstruction together with articles describing in depth the implementations used for the various imaging regimes. The section concludes with some theoretical references relating to the computer modelling of NMR image reconstruction and the development of new reconstruction schemes.

Barrett H H and Swindell W 1981 Computed Tomography *Radiological Imaging*, vol. 2, chapter 7 (New York: Academic Press) pp. 375–464

Shepp L A 1980 Computerised tomography and nuclear magnetic resonance *Journal of Computer Assisted Tomography* **4** 94–107

Cormack A M 1973 Reconstruction of densities from their projections, with applications in radiological physics *Physics in Medicine and Biology* **18** 195–207

Cormack A M 1963 Representation of a function by its line integrals, with some radiological applications *Journal of Applied Physics* **34** 2722–2727

Cormack A M 1964 Representation of a function by its line integrals, with some radiological applications II *Journal of Applied Physics* **35** 2908–2913

Mersereau R M 1976 Direct Fourier transform techniques in 3-D image reconstruction *Computers in Biology and Medicine* **6** 247–258

Shepp L A and Logan B F 1974 The Fourier reconstruction of a head section *IEEE Transactions on Nuclear Science* **NS-21** 21–32

Ljunggren S 1983 A simple graphical representation of Fourier-based imaging methods *Journal of Magnetic Resonance* **54** 338–343

Cho Z H 1974 General views on 3-D image reconstruction and computerised transverse axial tomography *IEEE Transactions on Nuclear Science* **NS-21** 44–71

Cho Z H and Burger J R 1977 Construction, restoration and enhancement of 2 and 3-dimensional images *IEEE Transactions on Nuclear Science* **NS-24** 886–899

Lai C.-M and Lauterbur P C 1981 The three-dimensional image reconstruction by nuclear magnetic resonance zeugmatography *Physics in Medicine and Biology* **26** 851–856

Tropper M M 1981 Image reconstruction for the NMR echo planar technique, and for a proposed adaptation to allow continuous data acquisition *Journal of Magnetic Resonance* **42** 193–202

Bangert V 1982 Nuclear magnetic resonance tomography, NMR scanner techniques and the theory of image reconstruction (PhD thesis) *VDI-Verlag GmbH, Dusseldorf*

Cho Z H, Hilal S K, Kim S H and Song H B 1983 Computer modelling and simulation of Fourier transform NMR imaging *Nuclear Magnetic Resonance (NMR) Imaging* eds C L Partain, A E James, F D Rollo and R R Price (Philadelphia: Saunders) pp. 453–486

Lai C M 1983 Reconstructing NMR images from projections under inhomogeneous magnetic field and non-linear field gradients *Physics in Medicine and Biology* **28** 925–938

Cho Z H (ed.) 1980 Development of methods and algorithms and Fourier transform nuclear magnetic resonance (NMR) tomographic imaging *ISS Lab Report No. 2* (Imaging System Science Laboratory, Dept of Electrical Science, Korea Advanced Institute of Science, Seoul, Korea)

Jeong J C, Song H B and Cho Z H 1982 Direct Fourier transform 3-D image reconstruction with modified concentric square sampling—application to NMR tomography *ISS Lab. Report No. 3* (Imaging System Science Laboratory, Dept. of Electrical Science, Korea Advanced Institute of Science, Seoul, Korea) pp. 161–197

Twieg D B 1983 The k-trajectory formulation of the NMR imaging process with applications in analysis and synthesis of imaging methods *Medical Physics* **10** 610–621

Sekihara K, Kuroda M and Kohno H 1984 Image restoration from non-uniform magnetic field influence for direct Fourier NMR imaging *Physics in Medicine and Biology* **29** 15–24

King K F and Moran P R 1984 A unified description of NMR imaging, data collection strategies and reconstruction *Medical Physics* **11** 1–14

8.6. Technical and engineering aspects of NMR imaging

Practical implementation has brought with it numerous problems which have had to be overcome. An understanding of such problems, and their solutions, is important in gaining an understanding of the workings and limitations of imaging systems, in addition to which the many ingenious technological developments are interesting in their own right.

This section contains a set of references ranging from basic system engineering descriptions of complete imaging systems to more detailed discussions of individual system components, such as gradient and RF coils, magnet technology, and so on.

Holland G N 1983 Systems engineering of a whole body proton magnetic resonance imaging system *Nuclear Magnetic Resonance (NMR) Imaging* eds C L Partain, A E James, F D Rollo and R R Price (Philadelphia: Saunders) pp. 128–151

Bottomley P A 1981 Instrumentation for whole-body NMR imaging *Proceedings of an International Symposium on Nuclear Magnetic Resonance Imaging, Winston-Salem, North Carolina, USA* (Bowman Gray School of Medicine Press) pp. 25–31

Johnson G, Hutchison J M S and Eastwood L M 1982 Instrumentation for NMR spin-warp imaging *Journal of Physics E: Scientific Instruments* **15** 74–79

Thomas S R, Ackerman J L, Goebel J R, Davis M, Kereiakes J G and Lin Y-Y 1982 Nuclear magnetic resonance imaging techniques as developed modestly within a university medical centre environment: What can the small system contribute at this point? *Magnetic Resonance Imaging* **1** 11–21

Roos C E, Caffey H T and Effersen K R 1983 Superconducting magnets *Nuclear Magnetic Resonance (NMR) Imaging* eds C L Partain, A E James, F D Rollo and R R Price (Philadelphia: Saunders) pp. 115–127

Hanley P 1981 Superconducting and resistive magnets in NMR scanning *Proceedings of an International Symposium on Nuclear Magnetic Resonance Imaging, Winston-Salem, North Carolina, USA* (Bowman Gray School of Medicine Press) pp. 41–49

Edelstein W A, Bottomley P A, Hart H R, Leue W M, Schenck J F and Redington R W 1981 NMR imaging at 5.1 MHz: Work in progress *Proceedings of an International Symposium on Nuclear Magnetic Resonance Imaging, Winston-Salem, North Carolina, USA* (Bowman Gray School of Medicine Press) pp. 139–145

Herman G T, Udupa J K, Kramer D M, Lauterbur P C, Rudin A M and Scheider J S 1981 Three-dimensional display of nuclear magnetic resonance images *Proceedings of the Society of Photo-Optical Instrumentation Engineers: Application of Optical Instrumentation in Medicine IX* **273** 35–40

Axel L, Herman G T, Udupa J K, Bottomley P A and Edelstein W A 1983 Three-dimensional display of nuclear magnetic resonance (NMR) cardiovascular images *Journal of Computer Assisted Tomography* **7** 172–174

GEC 1982 *NMR Site Planning Considerations* (General Electric Company, Milwaukee, Wisconsin, USA)

Ross R J, Thompson J S, Kim K and Bailey R A 1982 Site location and requirements for the installation of a nuclear magnetic resonance scanning unit *Magnetic Resonance Imaging* **1** 29–33

Hill H D W and Richards R E 1968 Limits of measurement in magnetic resonance *Journal of Physics E: Scientific Instruments* **1** 977–983

Hoult D I and Richards R E 1976 The signal-to-noise ratio of the nuclear magnetic resonance experiment *Journal of Magnetic Resonance* **24** 71–85

Freeman R and Hill H D W 1971 Phase and intensity anomalies in Fourier Transform NMR *Journal of Magnetic Resonance* **4** 366–383

Stejskal E O and Schaeffer J 1974 Comparisons of quadrature and single-phase Fourier Transform NMR *Journal of Magnetic Resonance* **14** 160–169

Hoult D I 1981 Radiofrequency coil technology in NMR scanning *Proceedings of an International Symposium on Nuclear Magnetic Resonance Imaging, Winston-Salem, North Carolina, USA* (Bowman Gray School of Medicine Press) pp. 33–39

Gadian D G and Robinson F N H 1979 Radiofrequency losses in NMR experiments on electrically conducting samples *Journal of Magnetic Resonance* **34** 449–455

Ginsberg D M and Melchner M J 1970 Optimum geometry of saddle shaped coils for generating a uniform magnetic field *Review of Scientific Instruments* **41** 122–123

Parker R S, Zupančič I and Pirš J 1973 Coil system to produce orthogonal linear magnetic field gradients *Journal of Physics E: Scientific Instruments* **6** 899–900

Bangert V and Mansfield P 1982 Magnetic field gradient coils for NMR imaging *Journal of Physics E: Scientific Instruments* **15** 235–239

Zupančič I 1962 Current shims for high-resolution nuclear magnetic resonance on the problem of correcting magnetic field inhomogeneities *Journal of Scientific Instruments* **39** 621–624

Hanley P E and Gordon R E 1981 The use of high-order gradients to vary the spatial extent of B_0 homogeneity in a high-resolution NMR experiment *Journal of Magnetic Resonance* **45** 520–524

Crooks L, Hoenninger J, Arakawa M, Watts J, McCarten B, Sheldon P, Kaufman L, Mills C M, Davis P L and Margulis A R 1984 High resolution magnetic resonance imaging: technical concepts and their implementations *Radiology* **151** 163–171
Redpath T W and Selbie R D 1984 A crossed-ellipse RF coil for NMR imaging of the head and neck *Physics in Medicine and Biology* **29** 739–744

8.7. Safety of NMR imaging

Safety considerations surrounding the clinical application of NMR imaging have attracted much attention. This has ranged from studies of the influence of NMR scanners on heart pacemakers and surgical prostheses to biological studies of the genetic effects of imaging exposure. A selection of the relevant publications is presented here.

Budinger T F 1981 Nuclear magnetic resonance (NMR) in vivo studies: known thresholds for health effects *Journal of Computer Assisted Tomography* **5** 800–811
Saunders R D and Orr J S 1983 Biological effects of NMR *Nuclear Magnetic Resonance (NMR) Imaging* eds C L Partain, A E James, F D Rollo and R R Price (Philadelphia: Saunders) pp. 383–396
Saunders R D 1981 Biological hazards of NMR *Proceedings of an International Symposium on Nuclear Magnetic Resonance Imaging, Winston-Salem, North Carolina, USA* (Bowman Gray School of Medicine Press) pp. 65–71
Budinger T F 1983 NMR in vivo studies: comparison with other non-invasive imaging techniques *Nuclear Magnetic Resonance (NMR) Imaging* eds C L Partain, A E James, F D Rollo and R R Price (Philadelphia: Saunders) pp. 357–374
Reid A, Smith F W and Hutchison J M S 1982 Nuclear magnetic resonance imaging and its safety implications: follow up of 181 patients *British Journal of Radiology* **55** 784–786
Pavlicek W, Geisinger M, Castle L, Barkowski G P, Meaney T F, Bream B L and Gallagher J H 1983 The effects of nuclear magnetic resonance on patients with cardiac pacemakers *Radiology* **147** 149–153
Davis P, Crooks L, Arakawa N, McRee R, Kaufman L and Margulis A R 1981 Potential hazards in nuclear magnetic resonance (NMR) imaging: heating effects of changing magnetic fields and r.f. fields on small metallic implants *Proceedings of the Society of Photo-Optical Instrumentation Engineers: Application of Optical Instrumentation in Medicine IX* **273** 210–214
New P F J, Rosen B R, Brady T J, Buonanno F S, Kistler J P, Burt C T, Hinshaw W S, Pohost G M and Taveras J M 1983 Potential hazards and artefacts of ferromagnetic and non-ferromagnetic surgical and dental materials and devices in nuclear magnetic resonance imaging *Radiology* **147** 139–148
Gore J C, McDonnell M J, Pennock J M and Stanbrook H S 1982 An assessment of the safety of rapidly changing magnetic fields in the rabbit: implications for NMR imaging *Magnetic Resonance Imaging* **1** 191–195
National Radiological Protection Board 1981 Exposure to nuclear magnetic resonance clinical imaging *Radiography* **47** 258–260
Bottomley P A and Edelstein W A 1981 Power deposition in whole-body NMR imaging *Medical Physics* **8** 510–512
Bottomley P A and Andrew E R 1978 RF magnetic field penetration, phase shift and power dissipation in biological tissue: implications for NMR imaging *Physics in Medicine and Biology* **23** 630–643
Thomas A and Morris P G 1981 The effects of NMR exposure on living organisms. I. A microbial assay *British Journal of Radiology* **54** 615–621

Cooke P and Morris P G 1981 The effect of NMR exposure on living organisms. II. A genetic study of human lymphocytes *British Journal of Radiology* **54** 622–625

Wolff S, Crooks L E, Brown P, Howard R and Painter R B 1980 Tests for DNA and chromosomal damage induced by nuclear magnetic resonance imaging *Radiology* **136** 707–710

Barnothy M F 1964 *Biological Effects of Magnetic Fields* vol. I and II (New York: Plenum Press)

8.8. NMR phantoms—image analysis and quantitation

In addition to quality assurance requirements, the potential of NMR as a quantitative modality has also resulted in interest in image analysis for NMR, and in the associated subject of NMR phantom development. The literature is sparse as yet. This selection from the available literature indicates some of the current problems, together with some proposed solutions.

Runge V M, Johnson G, Smith F W, Erickson J J, Price R R, Partain C L and James A E 1984 NMR phantom design: evaluation of performance parameters *Noninvasive Medical Imaging* **1** 49–60

Schneiders N J, Bryan R N and Willcott M R 1983 Phantoms for NMR image analysis *Nuclear Magnetic Resonance (NMR) Imaging* eds C L Partain, A E James, F D Rollo and R R Price (Philadelphia: Saunders) pp. 436–445

Lerski R A, Straughan K and Orr J S 1984 Calibration of proton density measurements in nuclear magnetic resonance imaging *Physics in Medicine and Biology* **29** 271–276

Pykett I L, Rosen B R, Buonanno F S and Brady T J 1983 Measurement of spin-lattice relaxation times in nuclear magnetic resonance imaging *Physics in Medicine and Biology* **28** 723–729

Redpath T W 1982 Calibration of the Aberdeen NMR imager for proton spin-lattice relaxation time measurements in vivo *Physics in Medicine and Biology* **27** 1057–1065

Schneiders N J 1983 Accurate T_2 NMR images *Medical Physics* **10** 642–645

Reisse J, Wilputte L and Zimmerman D 1983 NMR imaging: T_1 measurements and calibration in relation to so-called T_1 images *Annali deli' Istituto Superiore di Sanità* **19**(1) 51–56

Bakker C J G and Vriend J 1984 Multi-exponential water proton spin-lattice relaxation in biological tissues and its implications for quantitative NMR imaging *Physics in Medicine and Biology* **29** 509–518

Edelstein W A, Bottomley P A and Pfeifer L M 1984 A signal-to-noise calibration procedure for NMR imaging systems *Medical Physics* **11** 180–185

Rosen B R, Pykett I L and Brady T J 1984 Spin–lattice relaxation time measurements in two-dimensional nuclear magnetic resonance imaging: correction for plane selection and pulse sequence *Journal of Computer Assisted Tomography* **8** 195–199

8.9. NMR contrast agents

The intrinsically high contrast levels possible in NMR images have resulted in many non-invasive investigations being possible with NMR which would have required the administration of a contrast agent in other imaging modalities. This fact is frequently cited as an important advantage of NMR over x-ray CT. In spite of this, there is a growing area of research devoted to the development of NMR contrast agents to enhance further the diagnostic capabilities of NMR: however, there is very little yet published. A selection of review articles and recent research papers is presented here as an indication of the lines of study being pursued.

Brasch R C 1983 Methods of contrast enhancement for NMR imaging and potential applications *Radiology* **147** 781–788

Gore J C, Doyle F H and Pennock J M 1983 Relaxation rate enhancement observed in vivo by NMR imaging *Nuclear Magnetic Resonance (NMR) Imaging* eds C L Partain, A E James, F D Rollo and R R Price (Philadelphia: Saunders) pp. 94–106

Young I R, Clarke G J, Bailes D R, Pennock J M, Doyle F H and Bydder G M 1981 Enhancement of relaxation rate with paramagnetic contrast agents in NMR imaging *CT: the Journal of Computed Tomography* **5** 543–547

Chiarotti G, Christiani G and Giulotto L 1955 Proton relaxation in pure liquids and in liquids containing paramagnetic gases in solution *Nuovo Cimento* **1** 863–872

Lauterbur P C, Dias M H M and Rudin A M 1978 Augmentation of tissue water proton spin-lattice relaxation rate by in vivo addition of paramagnetic ions *Frontiers of Biological Energetics* **1** 752–759

Brady T J, Goldman M R, Pykett I L, Buonanno F S, Kistler J P, Newhouse J H, Burt C T, Hinshaw W S and Pohcot G M 1982 Proton nuclear magnetic resonance imaging of regionally ischaemic canine hearts: effect of paramagnetic proton signal enhancement *Radiology* **144** 343–347

Brasch R C, Nitecki D E, Brant-Zawadzki M, Enzmann D R, Wesbey G E, Tozer T N, Tuck L D, Cann C E, Fike V R and Sheldon P 1983 Brain nuclear magnetic resonance imaging enhanced by a paramagnetic nitroxide contrast agent: preliminary report *American Journal of Roentgenology* **141** 1019–1023

Runge V M, Stewart R E, Clanton J A, Jones M M, Lukehart C M, Partain C L and James A E 1983 Potential oral and intravenous paramagnetic NMR contrast agents *Radiology* **147** 789–791

Carr D H, Brown J H, Leung A W L and Pennock J M 1984 Iron and gadolinium chelates as contrast agents in NMR imaging: preliminary studies *Journal of Computer Assisted Tomography* **8** 385–389

8.10. Measurement of blood flow and oxygenation by NMR

NMR has long been used to study fluid flow, and many practical techniques for accurate measurement have been developed. Following the advent of imaging, there has been much interest in adapting these techniques for *in vivo* flow measurements. In addition, the paramagnetic properties of dissolved molecular oxygen can be used to determine blood P_{O_2} levels *in vivo*. This section contains a series of relevant articles.

Battocletti J H, Halbach R E, Salles-Cunha S X and Sances A 1981 The NMR blood flowmeter—theory and history *Medical Physics* **8** 435–443

Halbach R E, Battocletti J H, Salles-Cunha S X and Sances A 1981 The NMR blood flowmeter—design *Medical Physics* **8** 444–451

Salles-Cunha S X, Halbach R E, Battocletti J H and Sances A 1981 The NMR blood flowmeter—applications *Medical Physics* **8** 452–458

Singer J R 1959 Blood flow rates by nuclear magnetic resonance measurements *Science* **130** 1652–1653

Singer J R 1980 Blood flow measurements by NMR of the intact body *IEEE Transactions on Nuclear Sciences* **NS-27** 1245–1249

Morse O C and Singer J R 1970 Blood velocity measurements in intact subjects *Science* **170** 440–441

Radda G K, Styles P, Thulborn K R and Waterton J C 1981 A simple method of flow measurement by pulsed NMR *Journal of Magnetic Resonance* **42** 488–490

Grant J P and Back C 1982 NMR rheotomography: Feasibility and clinical potential *Medical Physics* **9** 188–193

Thulborn K R, Waterton J C and Radda G K 1981 Proton imaging for in vivo blood flow and oxygen consumption measurements *Journal of Magnetic Resonance* **45** 188–191

Bergmann W H 1983 A new approach to NMR flow imaging and analysis *Nuclear Magnetic Resonance (NMR) Imaging* eds C L Partain, A E James, F D Rollo and R R Price (Philadelphia: Saunders) pp. 487–493

Moran P R 1982 A flow velocity zeugmatographic interface for NMR imaging in humans *Magnetic Resonance Imaging* **1** 197–203

Hemminga M A, De Jager P A and Sonneveld A 1977 The study of flow by pulsed nuclear magnetic resonance. I. Measurement of flow rates in the presence of a stationary phase using a difference method *Journal of Magnetic Resonance* **27** 359–370

Hemminga M A and De Jager P A 1980 The study of flow by pulsed nuclear magnetic resonance. II. Measurement of flow velocities using a repetitive pulse method *Journal of Magnetic Resonance* **37** 1–16

Battocletti J H, Linehan J H, Larson S J, Sances A, Bowman R L, Kudravcev V, Genthe W K, Halbach R E and Evans S M 1972 Analysis of a nuclear magnetic resonance blood flowmeter for pulsatile flow *IEEE Transactions on Biomedical Engineering* **BME-19** 403–407

Devine R A B, Clarke L P, Vaughan S and Serafini A 1982 Theoretical analysis of the two-coil method for measuring fluid flow using nuclear magnetic resonance *Medical Physics* **9** 668–672

Thulborn K R, Waterton J C, Styles P and Radda G K 1981 Rapid measurement of blood oxygenation and flow by high-field ^{1}H n.m.r. *Biochemical Society Transactions* **9** 233–234

Jones D W and Child T F 1976 NMR in flowing systems *Advances in Magnetic Resonance* **8** 123–148

Singer J R 1978 NMR diffusion and flow measurements and an introduction to spin phase graphing *Journal of Physics E: Scientific Instruments* **11** 281–291

Brooks R A, Battocletti J H, Sances A, Larson S J, Bowman R L and Kudravcev V 1975 Nuclear magnetic relaxation in blood *IEEE Transactions on Biomedical Engineering* **BME-22** 12–17

Thulborn K R, Waterton J C, Matthews P M and Radda G K 1982 Oxygenation dependence of the transverse relaxation time of water protons in whole blood of high field *Biochimica et Biophysica Acta* **714** 265–270

George C R, Jacobs G, MacIntyre, W J, Lorig R J, Go R T, Nose Y and Meaney T F 1984 Magnetic resonance signal intensity patterns obtained from continuous and pulsatile flow methods *Radiology* **151** 421–428

8.11. NMR properties of biological tissue

NMR relaxation studies of biological tissue and of the state of the water in such tissues have been conducted for many years and there is a considerable volume of associated literature. But, in spite of the large amount of data available, controversy still persists over the interpretation of the results in terms of the dynamics of the tissue water. An understanding, at least in part, of the NMR response of tissue water is important for a complete understanding of NMR image content.

Much of this research has concentrated on the more simple biological substances, such as protein solutions, although there exists considerable published data relating to whole tissues, such as muscle. In addition, the majority of these experiments have been performed at high NMR frequencies relative to those typically used in imaging experiments) and, until recently, most of this work was performed *in vitro*. Following the advent of imaging, however, these investigations have been extended by many workers to consider the NMR properties of whole biological tissues, *in vivo* at imaging frequencies.

Presented here are references chosen to cover both the basic biophysical *in vitro* studies and the more applied *in vivo* imaging investigations. It is hoped that they will convey an impression of the current trends of thought (including the controversies) and allow an understanding of some of the factors pertinent to the interpretation of NMR image content.

Taylor D G and Bore C F 1981 A review of the magnetic resonance response of biological tissue and its applicability to the diagnosis of cancer by NMR radiology *CT: the Journal of Computed Tomography* **5** 122–133

Podo F and Orr J S (eds) 1983 EEC Workshop: Identification and characterisation of biological tissue by NMR *Annali dell' Istituto Superiore di Sanità* **19**(1)

Damadian R (ed) 1981 *NMR in Medicine* (Vol. 19 of *NMR Basic Principles and Progress* eds P Diehl, E Fluck and R Kasfeld) (Berlin: Springer-Verlag)

Damadian R, Zaner K, Hor D, DiMaio T, Minkoff L and Goldsmith M 1973 Nuclear magnetic resonance as a new tool in cancer research: human tumours by NMR *Annals of the New York Academy of Sciences* **222** 1048–1074

Koutcher J A, Goldsmith M and Damadian R 1978 NMR in cancer. X. A malignancy index to discriminate normal and cancerous tissue *Cancer* **41** 174–182

Damadian R 1971 Tumour detection by nuclear magnetic resonance *Science* **171** 1151–1153

Bryant R G and Halle B 1982 NMR relaxation of water in heterogeneous systems—consensus views? *Biophysics of Water* ed. F Franks (Chichester: John Wiley) pp. 389–393

Derbyshire W 1982 Dynamics of water in cellular systems *Biophysics of Water* ed. F Franks (Chichester: John Wiley) pp. 249–253

Mathur-De Vré R 1979 The NMR studies of water in biological systems *Progress in Biophysics and Molecular Biology* **35** 103–134

Shporer M and Civan M M 1977 The state of water and alkali cations within the intracellular fluids: the contribution of NMR spectroscopy *Current Topics in Membranes and Transport* **9** 1–69

Fullerton G D, Potter J L and Dornbluth N C 1982 NMR relaxation of protons in tissues and other macromolecular water solutions *Magnetic Resonance Imaging* **1** 209–228

Ahmad S B, Packer K J and Ramsden J M 1977 The dynamics of water in heterogeneous systems. II. Nuclear magnetic relaxation of the protons and deuterons of water molecules in a system with identically oriented planar interfaces *Molecular Physics* **33** 857–874

Zimmerman J R and Brittin W E 1957 Nuclear magnetic resonance studies in multiple phase systems: Lifetime of a water molecule in an absorbing phase on silica gel *Journal of Physical Chemistry* **6** 1328–1333

Pearson R T, Duff I D, Derbyshire W and Blanshard J M V 1974 An NMR investigation of rigor in porcine muscle *Biochimica et Biophysica Acta* **362** 188–200

Belton P S, Jackson R R and Packer K J 1972 Pulsed NMR studies of water in striated muscle. I. Transverse nuclear spin relaxation times and freezing effects *Biochimica et Biophysica Acta* **286** 16–25

Belton P S, Packer K J and Sellwood T C 1973 Pulsed NMR studies of water in striated muscle. II. Spin-lattice relaxation times and the dynamics of the non-freezing fraction of water *Biochimica et Biophysica Acta* **304** 56–64

Belton P S and Packer K J 1974 Pulsed NMR studies of water in striated muscle. III. The effect of water content *Biochimica et Biophysica Acta* **354** 305–314

Kasturi S R, Ranade S S and Shah S S 1976 Tissue hydration of malignant and uninvolved human tissues and its relevance to proton, spin-lattice relaxation mechanism *Proceedings of the Indian Academy of Science* **84**B 60–74

Ling C R, Foster M A and Mallard J R 1979 Changes in NMR relaxation times of adjacent muscle after implantation of malignant and normal tissue *British Journal of Cancer* **40** 898–902

Ling C R, Foster M A and Hutchison J M S 1980 Comparison of NMR water proton T_1 relaxation times of rabbit tissues at 24 MHz and 2.5 MHz *Physics in Medicine and Biology* **25** 748–751

Williams E S, Kaplan J I, Thatcher F, Zimmerman G and Knoebel S B 1980 Prolongation of proton spin-lattice relaxation times in regionally ischaemic tissue from dog hearts *Journal of Nuclear Medicine* **21** 449–453

Herfkens R, Davis P, Crooks L, Kaufman L, Price D, Miller T, Margulis A R, Watts J, Hoenninger J, Arakawa M and McRee R 1981 Nuclear magnetic resonance imaging of the abnormal live rat and correlations with tissue characteristics *Radiology* **141** 211–218

Fullerton G D, Cameron I L and Ord V A 1984 Frequency dependence of magnetic resonance spin-lattice relaxation of protons in biological materials *Radiology* **151** 135–138

Kimmich R, Nusser W and Winter F 1984 *In vivo* NMR field-cycling relaxation spectroscopy reveals $^{14}N^1H$ relaxation sinks in backbones of proteins *Physics in Medicine and Biology* **29** 593–596

8.12. ^{31}P NMR—topical magnetic resonance

The application of NMR to the study of phosphorus metabolites *in vivo* has aroused considerable clinical interest. This topical magnetic resonance (TMR) method provides complementary information to that available from NMR images and consequently there has been much effort on the part of commercial laboratories to combine TMR and imaging modalities in the one machine. Formidable technical problems are encountered when trying to do this.

This particular application of NMR has been separately treated in this book, but a limited bibliography is also included here. A series of review and research papers is presented which describe the theory and practical implementation of this technique. Several papers are cited which discuss the potential of chemical shift imaging.

Shaw D 1983 In vivo topical magnetic resonance *Nuclear Magnetic Resonance (NMR) Imaging* eds C L Partain, A E James, F D Rollo and R R Price (Philadelphia: Saunders) pp. 152–167

Gadian D G 1982 *Nuclear Magnetic Resonance and its Applications to Living Systems* (Oxford: Clarendon Press)

Gordon R E, Hanley P E and Shaw D 1982 Topical Magnetic Resonance *Progress in Nuclear Magnetic Resonance Spectroscopy* **15** 1–47

Scott K N, Brooker H R and Fitzsimmons J R 1983 Phosphorus NMR: Potential application to diagnosis *Nuclear Magnetic Resonance (NMR) Imaging* eds C L Partain, A E James, F D Rollo and R R Price (Philadelphia: Saunders) pp. 416–425

Chance B, Eleff S, Leigh J S, Barlow C, Ligetti L and Gigulai L 1983 Phosphorus NMR *Nuclear Magnetic Resonance (NMR) Imaging* eds C L Partain, A E James, F D Rollo and R R Price (Philadelphia: Saunders) pp. 399–415

Wilcott M R, Cook J P, Ford J J and Martin G E 1983 NMR in chemistry. *Nuclear Magnetic Resonance (NMR) Imaging* eds C L Partain, A E James, F D Rollo and R R Price (Philadelphia: Saunders) pp. 45–59

Nunnally R L 1983 Phosphorus NMR: Diagnosis of myocardial infarction *Nuclear Magnetic Resonance (NMR) Imaging.* eds C L Partain, A E James, F D Rollo and R R Price (Philadelphia: Saunders) pp. 426–432

Willcott M R, Ford J J and Martin G E 1981 Nuclear magnetic resonance spectroscopy *Proceedings of an International Symposium on Nuclear Magnetic Resonance Imaging, Winston-Salem, North Carolina, USA* (Bowman Gray School of Medicine Press) pp. 5–14

Hollis D P 1980 Nuclear magnetic resonance of phosphorus in the perfused heart *IEEE Transactions on Nuclear Science* **NS-27** 1250–1254

Brown T R 1983 In vivo enzyme kinetics using magnetisation transfer NMR *Nuclear Magnetic Resonance (NMR) Imaging.* eds C L Partain, A E James, F D Rollo and R R Price (Philadelphia: Saunders) pp. 433–435

Radda G K, Chan L, Bore P B, Gadian D G, Ross B D, Styles P and Taylor D 1981 Clinical applications of ^{31}P NMR *Proceedings of an International Symposium on Nuclear Magnetic Resonance Imaging, Winston-Salem, North Carolina, USA* (Bowman Gray School of Medicine Press) pp. 159–169

Bendel P, Lai C-M and Lauterbur P C 1980 ^{31}P spectroscopic zeugmatography of phosphorus metabolites *Journal of Magnetic Resonance* **38** 343–356

Scott K N, Brooker H R, Fitzsimmons J R, Bennett H F and Hick R C 1982 Spatial localisation of ^{31}P nuclear magnetic resonance signal by the sensitive point method *Journal of Magnetic Resonance* **50** 339–364

Brown T R, Kincaid B M and Ugurbil K 1982 NMR chemical shift imaging in three dimensions (in vivo biochemistry/^{31}P imaging/metabolite mapping) *Proceedings of the National Academy of Science of the USA* **79** 3523–3526

Contributors

Dr G M Bydder

Senior Lecturer
Department of Diagnostic Radiology
Royal Postgraduate Medical School
Hammersmith Hospital
Du Cane Road
London W12 0HS
England

Mr E B Cady

Senior Physicist
Department of Medical Physics and
    Bio-Engineering
University College Hospital and Medical School
11–20 Capper Street
London WC1E 6AU
England

Mr D T Delpy

Principal Physicist
Department of Medical Physics and
    Bio-Engineering
University College Hospital and Medical School
11–20 Capper Street
London WC1E 6AU
England

Mr R Inamdar

Research Student
Department of Physics
University of Surrey
Guildford GU2 5XH
England

Dr R A Lerski

Principal Physicist
Department of Medical Physics
Hammersmith Hospital
Du Cane Road
London W12 0HS
England

Professor J R Mallard   Head of Department
                         Department of Bio-Medical Physics and
                             Bio-Engineering
                         University of Aberdeen
                         Foresterhill
                         Aberdeen AB9 2ZD
                         Scotland

Mr K Straughan   Physicist
                         Department of Medical Physics
                         Hammersmith Hospital
                         Du Cane Road
                         London W12 0HS
                         England

Dr D G Taylor   Lecturer
                         Department of Physics
                         University of Surrey
                         Guildford GU12 5XH
                         England

Dr W E Timms   Head of NMR Systems Department
                         Oxford Research Systems
                         Nuffield Way
                         Abingdon
                         Oxon OX14 1RY
                         England

Dr P S Tofts   Physicist
                         Department of Medical Physics and
                             Bio-Engineering
                         Faculty of Clinical Sciences
                         University College London
                         11–20 Capper Street
                         London WC1E 6JA
                         England

Dr W Vennart   Lecturer
                         Department of Physics
                         University of Exeter
                         Stocker Road
                         Exeter EX4 4QL
                         England